The REACH OUT
Caregiver Support
Program

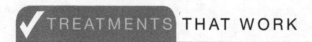

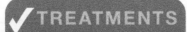
✔TREATMENTS THAT WORK

The REACH OUT Caregiver Support Program

A Skills Training Program for Caregivers of Persons with Dementia

CLINICIAN GUIDE

LOUIS D. BURGIO
Emeritus Professor, University of Alabama

MATTHEW J. WYNN
Washington University in St. Louis

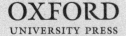

OXFORD
UNIVERSITY PRESS

OXFORD

UNIVERSITY PRESS

Oxford University Press is a department of the University of Oxford. It furthers
the University's objective of excellence in research, scholarship, and education
by publishing worldwide. Oxford is a registered trade mark of Oxford University
Press in the UK and certain other countries.

Published in the United States of America by Oxford University Press
198 Madison Avenue, New York, NY 10016, United States of America.

© Oxford University Press 2021

Library of Congress Cataloging-in-Publication Data
Names: Burgio, Louis D., editor. | Wynn, Matthew J., editor.
Title: The REACH OUT caregiver support program : a skills training program
for caregivers of persons with dementia : clinician guide /
[edited by] Louis D. Burgio, Matthew J. Wynn.
Description: 1 Edition. | New York : Oxford University Press, 2021. |
Includes bibliographical references and index. |
Identifiers: LCCN 2020047017 (print) | LCCN 2020047018 (ebook) |
ISBN 9780190855949 (hardback) | ISBN 9780190855963 (epub) |
ISBN 9780197506226
Subjects: LCSH: Caregivers—Services for. | Caregivers—Psychology. |
Stress management. | Dementia—Patients—Care.
Classification: LCC RA645.3 .R43 2021 (print) | LCC RA645.3 (ebook) |
DDC 362.1968/31—dc23
LC record available at https://lccn.loc.gov/2020047017
LC ebook record available at https://lccn.loc.gov/2020047018

DOI: 10.1093/med-psych/9780190855949.001.0001

9 8 7 6 5 4 3 2 1

Printed by Marquis, Canada

Stunning developments in health care have taken place over the last several years, but many of our widely accepted interventions and strategies in mental health and behavioral medicine have been brought into question by research evidence as not only lacking benefit, but perhaps, inducing harm (Barlow, 2010). Other strategies have been proven effective using the best current standards of evidence, resulting in broad-based recommendations to make these practices more available to the public (McHugh & Barlow, 2010). Several recent developments are behind this revolution. First, we have arrived at a much deeper understanding of pathology, both psychological and physical, which has led to the development of new, more precisely targeted interventions. Second, our research methodologies have improved substantially, such that we have reduced threats to internal and external validity, making the outcomes more directly applicable to clinical situations. Third, governments around the world and healthcare systems and policymakers have decided that the quality of care should improve, that it should be evidence based, and that it is in the public's interest to ensure that this happens (Barlow, 2004; Institute of Medicine, 2001, 2015; McHugh & Barlow, 2010).

Of course, the major stumbling block for clinicians everywhere is the accessibility of newly developed evidence-based psychological interventions. Workshops and books can go only so far in acquainting responsible and conscientious practitioners with the latest behavioral health care practices and their applicability to individual patients. This series, Treatments *ThatWork*™, is devoted to communicating these exciting new interventions to clinicians on the frontlines of practice.

The manuals and workbooks in this series contain step-by-step detailed procedures for assessing and treating specific problems and diagnoses. But this series goes beyond the books and manuals by providing ancillary materials that will approximate the supervisory process, thereby assisting practitioners in the implementation of these procedures in their practice.

In our emerging healthcare system, the growing consensus is that evidence-based practice offers the most responsible course of action for the mental health professional. All behavioral healthcare clinicians deeply desire to provide the best possible care for their patients. In this series, our aim is to close the dissemination and information gap and make that possible.

This Clinician Guide addresses the treatment of stress and burden experienced by caregivers for people with dementia. Clinicians will learn to utilize a tailored and flexible problem-solving protocol, examined and applied across a variety of clinical settings, and designed to be delivered across approximately six sessions. More than 16 million people in the United States provide informal, unpaid care to an adult and approximately one quarter of caregivers aged 60 or older support someone with a cognitive impairment. The guide is intended to be used by clinicians who are familiar with problem-solving approaches and who are comfortable tailoring the treatment to the caregiver's needs.

Because the processes and techniques that are presented here build upon a treatment protocol with extensive empirical support accumulated over three decades, *The REACH OUT Caregiver Support Program: A Skills Training Program for Caregivers of Persons with Dementia—Clinician Guide* will be an indispensable resource for all practitioners who wish to effectively and efficiently help caregivers of people with dementia reduce feelings of stress and burden and improve their quality of life.

David H. Barlow, Editor-in-Chief
Treatments *ThatWork*™
Boston, Massachusetts

References

Barlow, D. H. (2004). Psychological treatments. *American Psychologist, 59*, 869–878.

Barlow, D. H. (2010). Negative effects from psychological treatments: A perspective. *American Psychologist, 65*(2), 13–20.

Institute of Medicine. (2001). *Crossing the quality chasm: A new health system for the 21st century.* Washington, DC: National Academy Press.

Institute of Medicine. (2015). *Psychosocial interventions for mental and substance use disorders: A framework for establishing evidence-based standards.* Washington, DC: National Academies Press.

McHugh, R. K., & Barlow, D. H. (2010). Dissemination and implementation of evidence-based psychological interventions: A review of current efforts. *American Psychologist, 65*(2), 73–84.

Contents

Chapter 1   Development and Overview   *1*

Chapter 2   Risk Appraisal and Action Plans   *9*

Chapter 3   *Risk Area 1:* Home Safety   *25*

Chapter 4   *Risk Area 2:* Keeping the Caregiver Physically
Healthy   *29*

Chapter 5   *Risk Area 3:* Caregiver Emotional
Well-Being   *31*

Chapter 6   *Risk Area 4:* Managing Challenging
Behaviors   *41*

Chapter 7   *Risk Area 5:* Social Support   *51*

Chapter 8   Filling in the Gaps   *53*

APPENDICES
Appendix A   Caregiver Notebook   *57*

Appendix B   Generic Problem-Solving Form: Action Plan
Template   *87*

Appendix C   Sample Challenging Behavior Action
Plans   *89*

Appendix D   REACH OUT Home Safety Checklist   *105*

Appendix E   Healthy Lifestyle Guide   *109*

Appendix F   REACH OUT Pleasant Events Summary
Form   *115*

Appendix G   ABCs of Challenging Behaviors   *119*

Appendix H   Supplemental Material for Deciding Risk
Priority   *123*

Appendix I   Adverse Events   *127*

Appendix J   REACH OUT Clinician Treatment
Implementation and Tracking
Checklists   *131*

References   *137*

CHAPTER 1

Development and Overview

The development of REACH and REACH OUT

Our nation increasingly relies on family members or friends (i.e., informal caregivers) for needed care and support as we age. At present, caregiving for a loved one impacts one of every five American households. More than 16 million of us provide informal, unpaid care to an adult suffering from an illness or disability, enabling our loved ones to remain in their own homes and communities as long as possible (Alzheimer's Association, 2019). Because of our longer lifespans, a continued commitment to community-based care, and the tremendous value of informal home care, family caregiving is expected to become even more commonplace.

Family caregivers typically assume their caregiving role willingly and reap personal fulfillment from helping a family member, developing new skills, and strengthening family relationships. For these benefits, however, caregivers often sacrifice their own health and well-being. Depression, anxiety, poor physical health, and compromised immune function are more common among family caregivers than in adults not providing such care. In addition, the declining health of caregivers can compromise their ability to provide care to others (Dassel & Carr, 2014; Ma, Dorstyn, Ward, & Prentice, 2017).

The challenges and demands of caregiving are further compounded when the care recipient is cognitively impaired. Among caregivers of people aged 60 years or older, nearly one in four (about 26%) supports someone with a cognitive impairment, a memory problem, or a disorder such as Alzheimer's disease. Because these caregivers are relied upon to manage behavioral disturbances, attend to physical needs, and provide seemingly constant vigilance, they report higher levels of burden, stress, and depression than caregivers dealing with physical problems alone (Arthur, Gitlin, Kairalla, & Mann, 2018; Alzheimer's Association, 2019).

Recognizing the unique needs of family caregivers for people with dementia, the research community has been pursuing multiple avenues to identify effective interventions that support caregivers and improve their health and well-being. One of these evidence-based interventions, recently highlighted by the Institute of Medicine for implementation by public, private, and community organizations, is Resources for Enhancing Alzheimer's Caregiver Health, commonly referred to as REACH.

The REACH intervention is the result of two clinical trials sponsored by the National Institutes of Health (NIH). In the first trial (REACH I), initiated in 1995 by the National Institute on Aging (NIA) and National Institute for Nursing Research (NINR), each of six sites tested different strategies to help dementia caregivers manage the stress and burden of their caregiving roles. A quantitative analysis of results from the sites' collective five-year experience yielded a new intervention, which was subsequently tested across five sites in a randomized clinical trial (REACH II) and funded by NIH in 2001.

REACH II recognized the complexity of the problems causing caregiver stress and burden, and their tendency to vary in severity from one caregiver to another. To address these problems, research clinicians worked with caregivers to provide information, and most importantly multiple skills for managing the caregiving situation. REACH II included:

- education on dementia and caregiving;
- "active" skills training on techniques for pleasant events and relaxation;
- guidance in making the physical environment safer;
- and instruction and support for improved physical self-care, accessing social support, and a Behavior Problem Action Plan managing various limitations of Activities of Daily Living (ADL), Instrumental Activities of Daily Living (IADL), and behavior problems.

An initial Risk Appraisal shaped the order of intervention components and the intensity of their application.

The REACH II intervention was delivered over six months through as many as 12 in-home visits (some home visits could be substituted with therapeutic telephone sessions), interspersed with three therapeutic telephone sessions, and five support group sessions conducted with a specialized phone system. Findings showed significantly greater improvements in quality of life and depression in the intervention group (Belle et al., 2006).

Building on the success of these clinical trials, the next hurdle was to translate the REACH II intervention for feasible use in community-based settings. In 2004, the Administration on Aging accepted this challenge by awarding a grant to the Alabama Department of Senior Services to implement this intervention with four Area Agencies on Aging. Researchers from The University of Alabama partnered on the project, providing training and evaluation expertise as well as overall project guidance and management.

Consistent with procedures used in community-facilitated research, an advisory committee of key stakeholders participated in all design and delivery decisions to ensure full consideration of the realities of the healthcare and social environments. The eventual intervention product, termed REACH OUT (Resources for Enhancing Alzheimer's Caregiver Health: Offering Useful Treatments), was delivered to 272 dementia caregivers. This protocol reduced the number of treatment components (i.e., skills that were trained), required fewer intervention sessions, and shortened the overall length of the program. As with the earlier trials, the REACH OUT intervention resulted in significant positive changes in caregivers' stress and burden and in care recipient outcomes (Burgio et al., 2009).

The most recent iteration of REACH OUT is derived from a 1:1 pragmatic randomized clinical trial published in 2018 in the *Journal of the American Geriatrics Association* (Luchsinger et al., 2018). It compared the effectiveness of the REACH OUT program to the New York University Caregiver Intervention (NYUCI). Participants were 221 Hispanic caregivers who received either REACH OUT or the NYUCI intervention. The results showed that both interventions were equally effective in reducing caregiver burden (Luchsinger et al., 2018).

The REACH OUT training program was originally developed for use by Agency on Aging service providers, including social workers, nurses, and trained clinicians, and often delivered in caregivers' homes. Over the last several years, however, we have used the system successfully in primary care settings by using a combination of group and individual sessions with caregivers (Kessler et al., 2016). At this time, we can recommend its use in various primary care settings, including a clinician's office.

An overview of the REACH OUT intervention

In a nutshell, the REACH OUT intervention is multicomponent, tailored, and flexible. It is focused on the evidence-based therapeutic strategy of problem-solving. When possible, problem-solving should result in a written action plan. The intervention is delivered during six one-on-one sessions over a six-month period of time. All six sessions are intended to occur face-to-face between the caregiver and clinician; however, a maximum of two telephone sessions can be substituted for face-to-face sessions if necessary (usually as a result of logistical problems). These sessions can occur in the home; however, some or all the sessions can occur in the clinician's office or other primary care setting. Phone calls to caregivers should be scheduled to occur between one-on-one sessions to check on the caregiver's progress and make minor adjustments in Action Plans. These are referred to as "check-in calls."

The REACH studies showed that the causes of caregiver stress and burden are related to deficits in the caregiver's knowledge about dementia and the caregiving role. Most important, data showed that caregiver stress and burden revolved primarily around "five risk areas." These are:

- deficits in caregiver self-care and positive health behaviors
- low levels of caregiver emotional well-being
- inadequate social support
- home environments that produce detrimental effects in persons with dementia (PWD) and are possibly unsafe for both caregiver and care recipient
- the presence of care recipient problem behaviors

Thus, the REACH OUT intervention focuses its efforts on:

- improving the caregiver's knowledge about dementia and the caregiving role,
- improving knowledge and skills for physical and emotional well-being,
- optimizing the home environment for the care recipient,
- teaching the caregiver how to manage care recipient problem behaviors, and
- enhancing caregiver social support.

REACH OUT begins with a formal Risk Appraisal to determine how much emphasis to place on each of the intervention components. Thus, the intervention is standardized with respect to the number and types of treatment components but varies with respect to the dosing on individual treatment components. The tailoring of the intervention is guided by the findings of the risk appraisal. For example, caregivers with loved ones who do not display behavior problems will receive only a small dose of the intervention component designed to manage behavior problems (Behavior Management Action Plan). This enables the clinician to concentrate on those areas where risk factors are higher.

Tools to assist the clinician: Caregiver skills training and knowledge acquisition

The remainder of this guide contains the tools needed by the clinician to assist the caregiver in acquiring the knowledge and skills to become more effective in their role, and to reduce their level of stress and burden. The primary tool used to help caregivers acquire knowledge about dementia and the caregiving role is the Caregiver Notebook (see Appendix A). Provide each caregiver with a Notebook (typically a three-ring binder) that contains educational information about dementia, self-care, safety, and other relevant caregiver issues. The first section of the Caregiver Notebook should include copies of all subsequent Action Plans (Appendix B). It is a tool for organizing intervention materials and a resource guide for the caregiver to use during and after the intervention.

To identify and prioritize problem areas for each caregiver (i.e., "tailoring"), the councilor completes a risk appraisal (Chapter 2). The risk appraisal includes the 23-item REACH OUT Risk Appraisal Measure (RAM) and is supplemented by the 24-item Revised Memory and Behavior Problem Checklist (RMBPC).

Tailoring pertains to both the amount of clinician time spent in each risk module and the order of module presentation. The modules contain information and worksheets to assist you in enhancing the caregiver's knowledge of the five risk areas, and to form an Action Plan if the risk appraisal shows that the risk area is a priority for the caregiver. The five modules can be found in the guide in Chapters 3 through 7 and should be administered in an order tailored to the caregiver's needs and areas of risk.

You will use various forms to provide more effective treatment. These tools include, but are not limited to, a Home Safety Checklist (Appendix D), the Caregiver Guide for Healthy Living (Appendix E), the ABCs of behavior management (Appendix G), and, if indicated, Pleasant Events Training (Appendix F). These tools will be described later in this guide.

The most critical tool at the clinician's disposal is the Action Plan. It is important to understand that all aspects of the REACH OUT intervention involve *problem-solving* and the development of *written Action Plans* resulting from this process. The goal of this intervention is to engage the caregiver in joint problem-solving with the objective of creating written Action Plans targeting specific caregiving problems (e.g., improving caregiver health, addressing hazards in the physical environment, and managing challenging behaviors in care recipients). Problem-solving strategies are used to generate relevant information about the "target problems" and the overall caregiving situation, with special emphasis placed on the *context* in which the target problem occurs. In general, problem-solving should be thought of as a "mindset" or guiding strategy to use when working with the caregiver to develop and modify Action Plans over the intervention period. Sample Action Plans for common issues (e.g., bathroom accidents, communication difficulties) are provided in Appendix C.

Flow of intervention: Session-by-session description

The REACH OUT intervention is usually spread over a six-month period comprising six one-on-one sessions with the caregiver. If practical, check-in phone calls are interspersed between sessions. Table 1.1 is provided for reference. It is important to note that the presentation of material by session, as presented in this table, is only a sample. The actual order of presentation will be determined by the Risk Appraisal. We include Clinician Treatment Implementation and Tracking Checklists in Appendix J to assist you in applying this multicomponent intervention. These should be filled out following each session in order to help you adhere to the protocol and measure session-to-session caregiver progress. In Appendix H we provide supplemental material designed to help work through common barriers that may arise during the Risk Appraisal process. In Appendix I we present some common exigent circumstances or adverse events encountered during treatment sessions. This appendix includes the Geriatric Depression Scale that can be administered to caregivers if depression is suspected.

Session #1 is always dedicated to establishing rapport, introducing the REACH OUT program, providing psychoeducation regarding dementia or caregiving education, and completing the Risk Appraisal measures. If possible, attempt to do a safety walk-through early in the therapeutic process. This assessment can uncover risks that place the caregiver and care recipient at risk (e.g., loaded handguns, sharp objects).

Although you should provide at least some training on all five risk areas, not all risk areas will require an Action Plan. For example, if the care recipient is not displaying any challenging behaviors, or the caregiver is taking good care of their own health, there is no need for an Action Plan in these areas.

Table 1.1. Sample REACH OUT Intervention Schedule: 24 Weeks

One-On-One Sessions							
Intervention			Week				Total
Week	1	2–3	5–6	8–9	15–16	19–20	24
Session	1	2	3	4	5	6	6*

*Under extreme circumstances, a maximum of two of these sessions can be conducted via phone.

Sample Order of Topics Presented by Session

Week	Session	Check-In Phone Calls	Activities
1	#1		1. Greetings and establishing rapport 2. Describe the Program 3. Introduce Caregiver Notebook 4. Provide education about Alzheimer's disease, caregiving, patient/physician communication, anticipatory bereavement (refer to Caregiver Notebook) 5. Conduct Risk Appraisal
2		X (if session is scheduled for Week 3)	
2–3	#2		1. Introduce Action Plan #1 based on problem priority 2. Address questions 3. Introduce Home Safety and Conduct Home Safety Check
4		X	
5–6	#3		1. Follow up on Action Plan #1 2. Address questions 3. Introduce Action Plan #2 4. Discuss Problem Behaviors
7		X	
8–9	#4		1. Follow up on Action Plans #1 and #2 2. Address questions 3. Discuss caregiver health (Use the Caregiver Health Guide) 4. Introduce additional Action Plan if needed
12–13		X	
15–16	#5		1. Follow up on all Action Plans 2. Discuss Emotional Well-being: Stress and stress reduction (relaxation) or pleasant events 3. Provide Action Plan for stress reduction, relaxation technique, and/or pleasant events training
17–18		X	
19–20	#6		1. Follow up on all Action Plans 2. Discuss Enhancing Social Support 3. Introduce new Action Plan if needed 4. Address questions
22		X	

Note: The actual order of presentation will be determined by the Risk Appraisal

CHAPTER 2

Risk Appraisal and Action Plans

The Risk Appraisal: How to identify caregiver problems and prioritize them

The REACH OUT intervention combines psychoeducation and skills training within a problem-solving format. The first session is usually dedicated to providing caregivers with basic information about dementia, the trajectory of the disease, the caregiving role, and effects of stress and burden on caregivers' health. During the initial session caregivers will also learn the basic components of the REACH OUT intervention.

The content of the psychoeducational component can be found in the Caregiver Notebook (Appendix A). The notebook includes content and links to additional publicly accessible psychoeducational material. The skills that are taught during subsequent sessions focus on problem solving and creating Action Plans to address the five previous identified risk areas. Below, you will find detailed modules for these risk areas.

It should be noted that a standard Action Plan template is used for all the risk areas except Managing Challenging Behaviors and Pleasant Events Training. For these risk areas the ABCs of Behavior Management Form, and the Pleasant Events Training Form are used, respectively. You will note that these forms are merely topic-specific Action Plans.

To assess caregiver risk, we use the 23-item REACH OUT Risk Appraisal Measure (RAM; Burgio et al., 2009, Czaja et al., 2009), and the 24-item Revised Memory and Behavior Problem Checklist (RMBPC; Teri et al.,

1992). In prior research, we have found these tools to be sufficient for detecting the majority of caregiver issues. Information from these tools is used to help prioritize problem areas. Read the items on the checklist to the caregiver in an interview format.

Clinician Note

Information to be provided to caregivers (some of the appendices, worksheets, etc.) as well as items which you will need multiple copies of (e.g., assessments, clinician checklists) are available for download from the Treatments That Work website at www.oxfordclinicalpsych.com/ dementiacaregivers

---

The REACH OUT RAM—Risk Appraisal Measure

Caregiver Name:	Date:
Clinician Name:	Session or Check-in Phone Call Number:

Start the assessment by saying to the caregiver:

"Please answer the following questions about your [fill-in with how you want to refer to the caregiving situation and the term you want to use to refer to the care recipient]."

1. Do you have written information about memory loss, Alzheimer's disease, or dementia?
No   Yes   Unknown   Refused

2. Do you have a Living Will for [care recipient]?
No   Yes   Unknown   Refused

3. Do you or a family member have a Durable Power of Attorney or Guardianship for [care recipient]?
No   Yes   Unknown   Refused

4. Does [care recipient] have access to dangerous objects (e.g., gun, knife, or other sharp objects)?
No   Yes   Unknown   Refused

5. Does [care recipient] drive?
No   Yes   Unknown   Refused

6. Does [care recipient] smoke when alone in the house?
No   Yes   Unknown   Refused

7. Do you ever leave [care recipient] alone or unsupervised in the home?
No   Yes   Unknown   Refused

8. Does [care recipient] try to leave the home and wander outside?
No   Yes   Unknown   Refused

9. In general, would you say your health is:
Excellent   Very Good   Good   Fair   Poor   Unknown   Refused

10. In the past month, have you had trouble falling asleep, staying asleep, or waking up too early in the morning?

Never   Sometimes   Often   Very Often   Unknown   Refused

11. During the past week, have you felt depressed [or "your spirits were down"]?

Never   Sometimes   Often   Very Often   Unknown   Refused

12. Have you cut back on your physical activities, such as exercise and walking, because of caregiving?

No   Yes   Unknown   Refused

13. In the past month, has it been difficult to eat healthy or well-balanced meals on a regular basis?

Never   Sometimes   Often   Very Often   Unknown   Refused

14. Do you feel stressed about caring for [care recipient] and trying to meet other responsibilities (work/family)?

Never   Sometimes   Often   Very Often   Unknown   Refused

15. Do you feel strained (or nervous) around [care recipient]?

Never   Sometimes   Often   Very Often   Unknown   Refused

16. Has providing help to [care recipient] made you feel good about yourself?

Never   Sometimes   Often   Very Often   Unknown   Refused

17. Overall, how satisfied have you been in the past month with the physical help you have received from family members, friends, or neighbors?

Never   Sometimes   Often   Very Often   Unknown   Refused

18. In the past month, how satisfied have you been with the support, comfort, interest, and concern you have received from others?

Never   Sometimes   Often   Very Often   Unknown   Refused

19. If you were unable to care for [care recipient] or yourself, do you have someone who would take over?

No   Yes   Unknown   Refused

20. Is it difficult or stressful for you to help [care recipient] with basic daily activities, such as bathing, changing clothes, brushing teeth, or shaving?

Never   Sometimes   Often   Very Often   Unknown   Refused

21. Is it difficult or stressful for you to help [care recipient] with toileting, including cleaning up after accidents?

Never   Sometimes   Often   Very Often   Unknown   Refused

22. Over the past six months, have you felt inclined to (or, "have you been tempted to") scream or yell at [care recipient] because of the way they behaved?

Never   Sometimes   Often   Very Often   Unknown   Refused

23. Over the past six months, have you had to keep yourself from yelling at or slapping [care recipient] because of the way they behaved?

Never   Sometimes   Often   Very Often   Unknown   Refused

List here any additional problems that may have come up during the interview:

FORM 2.2

The RMBPC—Revised Memory and Behavior Problem Checklist (Roth et al., 2003)

> *Say this to the caregiver:* "The following is a list of problems people with memory problems sometimes experience. Please indicate if any of these problems have occurred during the past month. If so, how much has this bothered or upset you when it happened?

Has the problem occurred in the past month?

(circle one)   No   Yes

How much has the problem bothered you?

0 = Not at all   1 = A little   2 = Moderately   3 = Very much   4 = Extremely

Please answer all of the questions for both occurrence/nonoccurrence and reaction.

Problem	Has It Occurred in Past Month?		Reaction: (0–4)
1. Asking the same question again and again	No	Yes	
2. Trouble remembering recent events (i.e., items in the newspaper or TV)	No	Yes	
3. Trouble remembering significant past events	No	Yes	
4. Losing or misplacing things	No	Yes	
5. Forgetting what day it is	No	Yes	
6. Starting, but not finishing things	No	Yes	
7. Difficulty concentrating on a task	No	Yes	
8. Destroying property	No	Yes	
9. Doing things that embarrass you	No	Yes	
10. Waking you or other family members at night	No	Yes	
11. Talking loudly and rapidly	No	Yes	
12. Appearing anxious or worried	No	Yes	
13. Engaging in behaviors that are potentially dangerous to self and others	No	Yes	
14. Threats to hurt oneself	No	Yes	
15. Threats to hurt others	No	Yes	
16. Aggressive to others verbally	No	Yes	
17. Appearing sad or depressed	No	Yes	
18. Expressing feelings of hopelessness or sadness about the future	No	Yes	
19. Crying and tearfulness	No	Yes	
20. Commenting about death of self or others	No	Yes	
21. Talking about feeling lonely	No	Yes	
22. Comments about feeling worthless or being a burden to others	No	Yes	
23. Comments about feeling like a failure, or not having any worthwhile accomplishments in life	No	Yes	
24. Arguing, irritability, and/or complaining	No	Yes	

The next step is to prioritize the order in which to address these problems, or risk areas, with the caregiver. A "quick and dirty"—yet effective—means of prioritizing problems identified during the Risk Appraisal is to review with the caregiver all of the identified risks and then simply ask, "Which of these issues is affecting your happiness (well-being, quality of life, etc.) the most?" Repeat this question so that a short-list of risk areas can be identified (e.g., "OK, which issue is causing you the second-most amount of stress or bother?").

Please list the caregiver's top three to five priorities according to the Risk Appraisal measures and/or as expressed by the caregiver during subsequent sessions

Risk Priority 1	
Risk Priority 2	
Risk Priority 3	
Risk Priority 4	
Risk Priority 5	

The goal of REACH OUT is for you, the clinician, to engage the caregiver in joint problem solving with the objective of creating formal Action Plans targeting specific caregiving problems. Problem-solving strategies are used to generate relevant information about the "target problem" (risk area) and the overall caregiving situation, with special emphasis placed on the *context* in which the target problem occurs. In general, problem solving should be thought of as a "mindset" or guiding strategy to use when working with the caregiver to develop and modify Action Plans over the intervention period. Problem solving requires you to follow a step-by-step process when working with caregivers.

> **Clinician Note**
> *Supplemental material for deciding risk priority has been developed by the REACH researchers and can be found in Appendix H. These guidelines can be helpful and are worth reviewing. It is important to note, however, that these guidelines have not been validated empirically and should not be considered an algorithm for prioritizing identified risks.*

Step #1: Define the problem, set goals, and gather information

The essential task at this point in the process is to specify a well-defined target problem that is described objectively. Formulate in words: (a) What is the specific problem being addressed? And (b) how will success be measured (setting goals)? Gather information relevant to the problem, the context of the problem, and the caregiver's feelings about and reactions to the problem.

Defining the problem is an important step in determining the caregiver's perceptions and feelings regarding the problem. This process helps to establish, for example, "Where is the caregiver coming from?" and "What are their feelings about the problem?" As a practical step, you will start formulating the definition of the problem by restating aloud what the caregiver is reporting. This step will require you to actively listen to the caregiver and will reassure them that you indeed are listening to them.

The result of this process is an objectively defined problem that both the caregiver and clinician consider to be the most appropriate focus of the Action Plan.

For example, "My [care recipient] is ornery" is not sufficient because it does not provide you with enough information to determine what to do to address the targeted problem. Upon probing, you can almost always get the caregiver to be more specific about what is meant by "ornery." For example, "ornery" might translate into, "He gives me a hard time when I try to dress him." This is better, but still not specific enough. A much better definition is, "My [care recipient] hits and verbally abuses me when I try to dress him." This allows you to target the problems of physical aggression and/or verbal abuse during assistance with personal care. A clear and objective definition of the problem should be written into Section 1 on the Action Plan template. (See Appendix B for the complete Action Plan template form and Appendix C for sample Action Plans.)

Box from Action Plan template:

Define the Problem:

Setting goals for how the target problem will change is also part of this initial step. Goal setting provides direction for the generation of possible solutions. Goals should provide a concrete, realistic expression of the caregiver's expectations. There are two general types of goals: (1) problem-focused and (2) emotion-focused. Problem-focused goals center on actual changes in the target problem. Emotion-focused goals are aimed at managing caregiver emotions or feelings that are linked to the targeted problem. It is not unusual for actual changes in the target problem to be difficult to achieve. Thus, changing the caregiver's feelings about the problem would be a worthwhile and necessary goal. A brief statement of the goal is placed in the second box on the Action Plan template.

Box from Action Plan template:

```
Goal of Action Plan:



```

Step #2: List possible solutions on a separate pad of paper

This step has also been termed "brainstorming," because the goal is to generate as many solutions as possible—regardless of their apparent feasibility. Work together with the caregiver to generate a list of all possible solutions or choices that could be made in response to the problem. Praise any response at this stage and assist by providing possible solutions. You and the caregiver are challenged to generate and record as many diverse solutions as possible without judging the feasibility or acceptability of the solution. Listing solutions without judging can be difficult. During this process, caregivers often will object to a possible solution with "yes, but . . ." statements. When possible, discourage the caregiver from criticizing or negating solutions until the next step. Be careful that your language does not encourage critical comments. For example, try not to use statements such as, "What do you think about . . .?" or "Do you think [solution] will work?" Initially, you may need to provide the caregiver with possible solutions or strategies. The goal is joint problem solving between you and the caregiver, so many possible solutions are generated with the hope that the caregiver will implement one or a combination of solutions, resulting in problem resolution or management.

Step #3: Decision-making and prescribing solutions to be used

After the brainstorming activity is completed, negotiate the solution(s) to be attempted with the caregiver. Allow the caregiver to express whether any of the solutions are "unacceptable" due to strong feelings about the nature of the solution (i.e., certain solutions listed can be ruled out). It is preferable to not give caregivers the opportunity to rule out strategies "they think will not work," or that "they have already tried." It is often necessary to encourage caregivers to try strategies that they do not believe in and/or strategies they have ineffectively implemented in the past. With assistance, many of these formerly ineffective strategies might be effective. Only rule out strategies the caregiver *refuses* to consider. Basically, the list of solutions will be refined to strategies with the greatest likelihood of implementation, utility, and success.

Step #4: Solution implementation and tracking progress toward stated goal

Develop the Action Plan with the caregiver. Write down the specific steps to the problem's solution on the Action Plan section below. Make sure the caregiver understands and is willing to try the identified strategies. Role play and demonstrate possible strategies whenever possible in the presentation of an Action Plan. At the very least, provide multiple examples of how the problem might manifest and present how the caregiver should respond. Assessment of the caregiver's implementation of Action Plan solutions and strategies and the caregiver's satisfaction with the Action Plan as well as necessary modifications will be done during the next session, or during a check-in phone call, if used.

Subsequent sessions should include the following:

- Assessment of the caregiver's use of the solutions and strategies outlined in the Action Plan,
- Evaluation of the usefulness and success of the solutions, and
- Praise for the caregiver's effort in trying/using solutions and strategies.

Box from Action Plan template:

Action Plan for Solving Problem:

1.

2.

3.

4.   ·

General Information:

You are a dedicated caregiver and you are doing a great job. We understand that this problem can be very upsetting to you and are committed to helping you with this problem. We believe these strategies will help and look forward to working with you in the coming weeks.

Points to keep in mind as the caregiver moves forward with the Action Plan:

- Customize the Action Plan by including information about the nature of the problem and highlighting recommended strategies.
- Use simple, easy-to-understand language (no jargon).
- Be mindful of the native language and literacy level of the caregiver.
- Be aware of any vision problems (e.g., use larger font).
- Use action words to begin the description of each strategy.
- Review target problem and discuss what "success" would look like to the caregiver (goal).
- Read the definition of the target problem aloud to make sure that you and the caregiver have a similar understanding of the problem.
- Most often the caregiver will agree with the definition of the target problem. From time to time, however, a caregiver may forget what was discussed in the previous session or may no longer agree. In this situation, if appropriate, discuss the discrepancy with the caregiver with the goal of bringing them back to the previously agreed upon target problem.
- Discuss what would make the caregiver feel better about this problem or what it would take for them to consider the problem resolved (e.g., having someone help out two afternoons per week). Make sure these goals are consistent with the goals defined in previous sessions.

- Remind the caregiver that the strategies listed in the Action Plan require *knowledge acquisition* and *frequent practice*. Explain that the process will unfold over the next several weeks as you work together on these and other strategies.
- Explain what an Action Plan is not (e.g., "I will not be asking you to try new medications or go out and buy a lot of things.") and what it is (e.g., "I will be talking to you more about things such as communicating better with [care recipient] and making changes in your living space to make caregiving easier and safer.")
- Encourage the caregiver to be open to new ideas and strategies.
- Describe your working relationship with the caregiver as a partnership in which you will continue to work together to refine and reshape ideas.
- Reiterate that we do things this way because we have worked with a lot of caregivers over the years and have found these strategies to work most often. Emphasize that many other initially reluctant caregivers also have found success using these strategies.
- Recognize that changes may feel awkward initially because the caregiver and care recipient have a long history of interacting in set ways. With practice, however, attempting these new strategies will become easier.

Step 5: Practice and provide feedback for each action plan

It is important that the caregiver practices and implements strategies or skills outlined in the Action Plan with you. It is important to offer encouragement and rationale to keep the caregiver engaged and motivated. Ask the caregiver to begin using the identified strategies immediately and to keep practicing until the next session. Encourage implementation by asking the caregiver to make a commitment to practice the Action Plan strategies and solutions daily (or as often as possible). Emphasize that things need to be tried repeatedly and consistently for them to be helpful. Try to express commitment to a working partnership by reminding the caregiver of the intervention timeline, pointing out that you will be working closely with them over the next several months. Finally, commit to revising Action Plans in order to find at least one strategy that works. If it is practical for you to be available by phone and/or e-mail, discuss how this would be done in your practice.

Language to consider:

- "It often helps to have someone watch what you are doing so you can remember what works and what is difficult."
- "Practicing with someone can help you find ways to improve."
- "Show me how you will carry out this strategy."
- "Let's go through the whole thing and talk about it afterward."

After the practice exercise is completed, highlight the good points and areas that need improvement. Then return to the specific steps with corrections before providing words of encouragement.

Language to consider:

- "I really liked the way you . . . [name the parts that went well]."
- "I have a few suggestions about how things might go better in certain places."
- "Can we try those parts again and try something a little different?"
- "I know this may be difficult at this time, but I do think these strategies will help, and I will be here to provide support and guidance."

Clinician Note
The Action Plan template is available in Appendix B, and sample Action Plans are available in Appendix C.

CHAPTER 3

Introducing safety issues to caregivers

Safety issues were one of the first risk areas considered in developing the original REACH project. As a person with dementia (PWD) moves to more advanced stages of the disease, maintaining personal safety becomes increasingly important. The effects of the disease can cause the PWD to do dangerous things. Each PWD is different; thus, it can be difficult to predict what type of safety problems will occur as the individual's disease progresses.

At this point, review the safety information and the REACH OUT Home Safety Checklist with the caregiver (in the Caregiver Notebook, Appendix A; the checklist is also included as Appendix D for you, the clinician).

Safety assessment

Safety assessments are conducted early in the therapeutic process. If practical in your setting, ask the caregiver for permission to conduct a safety walk-through of the home with the caregiver. Be sure to note positives and be sensitive in pointing out areas needing attention or improvement. Remember this is not a military inspection! The goal is to make changes that make things simpler, safer, and easier for the caregiver to manage.

Appendix D contains a Home Safety Checklist. If it is impractical for you to do a walk-through, review the assessment checklist with the caregiver and ask them to complete a walk-through on their own prior to the next appointment. Clinicians may note that not all items in the check-list will apply to every caregiver. It will be up to you and the caregiver to home in on the most relevant issues and problem-solve. Review the completed checklist during the next session. If responses on the form indicate areas wherein safety issues require improvement, the goal(s) should be incorporated into an Action Plan. Below is a list of common safety considerations for the home.

In the kitchen and bathroom

- Make the stove safe. Some electric stoves have a switch in the back that will make it impossible to turn the stove on. You can remove the knobs from gas or electric stoves or buy protective covers for knobs and burners.
- Unplug electrical appliances that remain in view, especially at night.
- Paint or otherwise mark hot water faucets to minimize confusion. Lower temperature of hot water heater to a safe level.
- Keep a working fire extinguisher in the kitchen.
- Put matches, lighters, and poisonous cleaners out of sight and reach.
- Cabinets may be secured by the plastic lock mechanisms people use to keep toddlers out of harm's way. Also, put knives behind secured cabinet doors.
- Have working smoke detectors in the house.
- Disable the lock on the inside of bathroom doors.
- Use nonslip strips in the tub and showers and use bathmats with nonskid backing.
- Install safety bars in bathroom.

Other living areas

- Do not have any weapons available.
- Obstruct hot surfaces such as radiators.
- Know and practice a fire escape route.
- Have adequate but not glaring lighting. Use night lights for safety.
- Stairs are dangerous! Use a "baby gate" at top and bottom and be sure stair rails are secure.

- Remove all clutter from steps.
- Secure all doors, including basement and back doors. You can set up an alarm system to alert you when they are opened. You can place locks very high or very low.
- It might be appropriate to lock windows or use guards that lock the window open at a safe height.
- Clear floors of clutter. Secure rugs from slipping or remove them.
- Placing reflector tape where the care recipient bumps into things can help. Rubber soles on shoes and slippers are less likely to slip.
- Remove poisonous houseplants.
- Have emergency numbers available by each phone. Include police, fire department, doctors' names and numbers, poison control center, and nearest reliable neighbor. Remember 911.
- Buy or prepare a first aid kit.

Periodic follow-up

At each contact, it is important to "check in" with caregivers regarding their implementation of the safety suggestions and to note if they find them beneficial. Emphasize that safety needs should be re-evaluated as the disease progresses.

CHAPTER 4

Risk Area 2: Keeping the Caregiver Physically Healthy

Physical well-being

Most outcomes in caregiver intervention research have focused on the mental health or psychosocial consequences of caregiving. However, caregiving can also negatively affect caregivers' physical health and health behaviors. Because caregiving can be a prolonged stressor, caregivers may be at risk for conditions such as high blood pressure and increased susceptibility to colds and flu. Caregivers also appear less likely than their noncaregiving counterparts to practice preventive health behaviors that are important in chronic disease prevention and control. Moreover, data show that older adults caring for a disabled spouse who experienced strain as a result of their caregiving role were 63% more likely to die than noncaregivers over a four-year observation period (Schulz & Beach, 1999). The result is that caregivers tend to neglect their own healthcare needs because they are so busy taking care of their loved ones. For the caregiver to be fully able to care for their loved ones with dementia, however, they must attend to their own health needs.

The REACH OUT intervention's physical well-being component focuses on basic education and referral to healthcare providers to maintain caregiver physical health. This chapter consists of reviewing the Healthy Lifestyle Guide, which is found in Appendix E and is included in the Caregiver Notebook (Appendix A). It is helpful to review the guide with the caregiver section by section. More specifically, during the session you might say "OK, I'll get you started," and then choose a section from the guide. We recommend starting with the section labeled, "Medical Care." You might say, "When was your last routine physical check-up?" (We have discovered that many caregivers have not had a routine checkup in years.) If the caregiver has not had a check-up recently, enter it as a goal of an Action Plan. Track the caregiver's progress toward this goal during check-in phone calls and subsequent sessions.

Periodic follow-up

At each subsequent session, it is important to check in with caregivers regarding any progress toward their healthcare goals. Encourage caregivers to make use of the guide and review entries at each session.

CHAPTER 5

Risk Area 3: Caregiver Emotional Well-Being

Rationale

The tasks and burdens associated with caregiving for a person with dementia are typically numerous and varied; in addition, they frequently change over the course of the disease. Given these often overwhelming responsibilities, caring for family members with dementia frequently is associated with increased levels of depression, stress, anxiety, and anger, along with a decrease in doing things that the caregiver found pleasing in their life. Thus, the well-being intervention components are designed to (1) decrease stress by teaching relaxation and (2) increase pleasant events.

Well-Being Strategy #1: *Inducing relaxation through Signal Breath**

We recommend teaching Signal Breath to all caregivers and also have included it in the Caregiver Notebook (Appendix A). The Signal Breath relaxation deep-breathing techniques help to circulate more oxygen throughout the body. Deep breathing has been shown to increase alertness and reduce the effects of stress. The Signal Breath technique is easy to learn. It was specifically designed for use in the middle of a stressful situation. We are aware that caregivers have very little "down time." We emphasize teaching Signal Breath because it only takes a few moments to do and can potentially reduce a lot of tension.

---

* *The Signal Breath technique was originally designed by Dr. Richard L. Hanson at the Long Beach VA Medical Center in his work with chronic pain patients and has been adapted for use with caregivers of persons with dementia by Jocelyn Shealy McGee, MSG, MA at the Palo Alto VA Health Care System.*

Instructions for Signal Breath

1. Ask the caregiver: "What sort of caregiving situations have been frustrating or stressful for you?" (Encourage the caregiver to name a couple of problems that have recently come up during caregiving.) "To help you reduce your stress and tension in situations such as these, we are going to practice a relaxation strategy called Signal Breath. I encourage you to use this strategy daily. Our goal in practicing this simple technique is to help you gain more control over your tension so that you can manage stressful situations better."

2. Say, "The Signal Breath technique was designed specifically to help you when you are in the middle of stressful situations. I chose this simple but effective technique because caregivers often have limited time for themselves. The great thing about the Signal Breath is that it only takes a moment to do and can potentially reduce a lot of tension. Also, it can be used anywhere, at any time, as many times as you want. In fact, you could even use the Signal Breath in a crowded room and no one would know."

3. "OK, so let's try this out. I want you to take in a deep breath and hold it for a few seconds. However, don't breathe so deeply or hold your breath so long that it is uncomfortable. About two or three seconds is usually long enough. Exhale slowly while at the same time saying calming words such as 'relax,' 'let go,' or 'easy does it' to yourself. Also, while you are exhaling, try to let your jaw, shoulders, and arms go loose and limp."

4. "Let's try it again. Take in a deep breath and hold it. Now, let it go slowly and say calming words to yourself. Let your jaw, shoulders, and arms go loose and limp."

5. "One more time, take in a deep breath and hold it. Let it out slowly. Relax. Let your body go loose and limp."

> **Clinician Note**
> *If the caregiver says the Signal Breath didn't work or it was not helpful, remind them that it requires regular practice, and encourage them to practice regularly.*

6. "I encourage you to practice the Signal Breath at least once—but preferably several times—a day. Caregivers often find it useful to practice when they are not stressed, because it helps reduce feelings of tension when stressful situations ultimately arise. But remember to practice it during a stressful situation, if possible."

Incorporate the Signal Breath strategy, as well as a suggested schedule of its use, into an Action Plan.

Periodic follow-up

During subsequent sessions, it is important to check in with caregivers regarding their use of Signal Breath and to note whether they find it beneficial. Encourage caregivers to practice Signal Breath at least daily and whenever they are feeling stressed or overwhelmed.

Well-Being Strategy #2: *Increasing pleasant events for the caregiver and for the dyad*

This section presents a protocol for helping caregivers increase the number of pleasant events in their lives. However, sometimes a caregiver-specific pleasant event is not possible, or the caregiver expresses a strong preference for a dyadic pleasant event. Pleasant events for the caregiver and for the dyad are discussed separately. Note that this protocol is applied using Form 5.1: Pleasant Events Action Plan Worksheet, shown later in this chapter. First, clinicians should use Form 5.1 to prompt ideas and begin a list of activities. Then, clinicians and caregivers fill out Form 5.2 together, including specifics about one of the items identified on Form 5.1. Finally, clinicians transfer the information from Form 5.2 to Appendix F (the REACH OUT Pleasant Events Summary Form) in order to make the information easier for the caregiver to follow and track throughout their week.

Increasing pleasant events for the caregiver

Criteria for using this protocol are met if items 10, 11, 14, and 22 are endorsed on the REACH OUT RAM—Risk Appraisal Measure (Form 2.1) or if you note obvious signs of dysphoria or depression. Note that this protocol can be triggered even if depression is not endorsed on the Risk Appraisal Measure. By engaging in pleasant events, caregivers may experience increased quality of life and social support, as well as improved physical and emotional health.

Sample script

1. "Although caregiving is time consuming, it is important that you take time to do things that you enjoy. This is important because if all your activities are limited to your caregiving responsibilities, you might begin feeling exhausted and frustrated."
2. "Depression or pervasive sadness can develop when we experience too many unpleasant events or too few pleasant events. As a caregiver, having too many unpleasant events and too few pleasant events can make you feel like you have no control. You may say to yourself, 'What is the use? It seems like there is nothing I can do to make things better.' You can feel better, however, by making sure your day includes at least a few events that you find pleasing."
3. "What counts as a pleasant event? Pleasant events do not have to be big activities that require a lot of planning. They can be small activities that you do on your own, with friends, or with your care recipient. Examples of pleasant events are reading, going for a walk, and listening to music. Even though these activities may last only 15 minutes, taking this time out for yourself is important for your well-being. Anything you like to do is a pleasant event!"

Remember the following key point: Start small and keep it simple! The most important thing to remember is to help caregivers choose events that they can do every day or a few times a week. Choosing small events (proximal goals) that do not require a lot of planning is the best way to start increasing pleasant events in caregivers' lives. The caregiver may enjoy traveling (distal goal), but realistically most caregivers cannot take a trip every day. Smaller and more realistic activities would be going on a day trip, going to the mall, or biking or walking around their neighborhood.

Clinician Note

If you ascertain that a distal goal, for example, visiting family who live out of town, is realistic you can use problem solving and an Action Plan to help the caregiver reach this goal. However, be sure to work on a couple of proximal pleasant events concurrently.

Clinician Note

Information to be provided to caregivers (some of the appendices, worksheets, etc.) as well as items which you will need multiple copies of (e.g., assessments, clinician checklists) are available for download from the Treatments That Work website at www.oxfordclinicalpsych.com/ dementiacaregivers

---

FORM 5.1
Pleasant Events Action Plan Worksheet (Part 1)

Use this worksheet during a pleasant events session. Begin by asking these questions:

- "Would you rather find pleasant events for yourself, or pleasant activities you can do with your _____.'"
- "Tell me about some things you find pleasurable."
- "Are there activities that you used to do and found pleasant but can't do any longer because you are caring for _____."

If the first three questions fail to produce pleasant events, say the following:

- "Here are examples of events you might find pleasurable. Let's review the list and see if any appeal to you."
  - Listening to music
  - Window shopping or buying something for yourself or someone special
  - Taking a walk
  - Reading
  - Going to a house of worship
  - Praying at home with prayer book
  - Going out to eat with friends or family members
  - Cooking or baking your favorite foods
  - Writing letters, cards
  - Doing crafts
  - Exercising
  - Going to the movies
  - Renting a video
  - Going for a car ride
  - Having a picnic in the park
  - Having friends over
  - Enjoying flowers
  - Gardening
  - Looking at the moon and stars
  - Taking a nap
  - Spending time with your children or grandchildren
  - Listening to the radio
  - Watching your favorite TV show
- "Let's work together to figure out pleasant events that you could do on a regular basis. Let's start by creating a list of possible activities." (Use the first page of the Summary Form.)

How to use the REACH OUT Pleasant Events Summary Form (Appendix F)

The REACH OUT Pleasant Events Summary Form (see Appendix F) is meant to supplement the Pleasant Events Action Plan. The form summarizes all the realistic pleasant events identified, it specifies which pleasant event is targeted for that week, and it outlines the schedule for the pleasant events for that week. Along with the caregiver, go through Form 5.2 to gather the information you will need to be able to complete the REACH OUT Pleasant Events Summary Form. To begin this form, say, "Now let's review your personal list of pleasant events and pick one activity that you would like to schedule during this session. Choose an activity that you believe you can realistically do this week."

FORM 5.2
Pleasant Events Action Plan Worksheet (Part 2)

The pleasant event I will be doing this week is:

_____

Now, fill in the following information for this activity. (Ask the caregiver to fill in the blanks or if preferred, you may fill in the blanks.)

1. I need the following materials: _____

_____

2. _____ will take place at the following location:

_____

3. When and how often can_____ be done?

_____

4. How much time will _____ take?

5. The steps I need to take in order to complete _____ are:

a. _____

b. _____

c. _____

d. _____

Based on your answers to these questions, let's schedule when you will be doing your pleasant event this week. (The clinician should distill this information onto the REACH OUT Pleasant Events Summary Form in Appendix F.)

The pleasant event I will be doing over the next couple of weeks is:

_____

I will do my pleasant event on the following day(s) and time(s):

_____

The completed REACH OUT Pleasant Events Summary Form (Appendix F) should be posted where you will see it every day (e.g., refrigerator, bedside table).

Home practice

Say: "Do the pleasant events you have chosen at the time(s) indicated on your schedule (use the summary form in Appendix F). We will review this at our next meeting."

Ask the caregiver the following questions:

- "Do you have any concerns about completing your pleasant event?"
- "In what we covered, what, if anything, is unclear?"
- "What other questions do you have about doing this?"

Say, "It is important that you try to do your pleasant activity this week. That is the only way to see how it really works. If you do not try it, we will not know whether it helps. I will be interested to hear all about how it went when I see you next time. I realize this might be difficult, but you are really working hard and need a break."

During the next session

Say, "I would like to review the materials you received during your last visit." (Review information from the REACH OUT Pleasant Events Summary Form.) "Did you complete your pleasant event?"

If caregiver did complete the home practice

Provide lots of praise and ask the caregiver the following questions:

- "How did you feel during your pleasant activity?"
- "How did you feel after you completed your pleasant activity?"
- "How did it feel to complete your goal?"

If caregiver did not complete the home practice

Analyze barriers to doing the pleasant event (i.e., "What stopped you from doing your pleasant activity?").

Pleasant events for you and your care recipient

Suggested script: "It is not always possible for you to do activities without [care recipient]. This can be difficult because you have so many tasks to do as a caregiver, but I believe it is valuable to continue to enjoy each other's company by doing enjoyable activities. We are now going to develop a list of pleasant events that you and your relative can enjoy together. Let's begin by reviewing Form 5.1 from before. Let's think of at least 10 events that you and your relative can enjoy together.

"From this list of activities, are there any that you believe you can do on a regular basis with [care recipient]? If so, write them down in Appendix F, in the section called, 'List of pleasant events for [care recipient] and me.' If there are events that you enjoy that are not on this list, please add them to the list. Remember, choose activities that you realistically can do on a daily or weekly basis.

"If you are having trouble coming up with possible activities, think about events you used to enjoy doing together in the past. Is it possible to still do those activities? If not, can they be modified? For example, if you used to take long walks together, you can now take short walks (one to two blocks) around your neighborhood.

"Remember to start small and keep it simple (e.g., give care recipient a hand massage, read to them, or listen to music together). The goal is to develop activities that you will enjoy together.

"Let's review Form 5.1 and pick an activity that you would like to schedule this week for you and your relative to enjoy together. Choose an activity that you believe you can realistically do together this week."

From this point on, you can follow the same procedures outlined above in the caregiver-only pleasant event protocol, including filling in information about the pleasant event on the REACH OUT Pleasant Event Summary Form, discussing home practice, and revisiting the pleasant event during the next session.

If caregiver did not do pleasant event with care recipient

Analyze barriers to completing the pleasant events. For example, ask, "What stopped you from doing the pleasant event with [care recipient]?"

CHAPTER 6

Risk Area 4: Managing Challenging Behaviors

The ABCs of behavior management

When using this strategy, gathering information about the context of challenging behavior is accomplished via the "ABC Process" (Teri et al., 1998). This is a variation on the problem-solving process discussed throughout this clinician guide. This process provides information about the antecedents and consequences of the target problem. To facilitate the development of an individualized Action Plan with the greatest likelihood of success, work with the caregiver to obtain relevant information regarding the context of the problem (e.g., information on the time of day, specific setting where the problem occurs, and what has been tried in the past). The ABCs of Challenging Behaviors worksheet (see Appendix G) structures this process for you, and you must be very familiar with this form before working with REACH OUT clients.

> **Clinician Note**
> *Information to be provided to caregivers (some of the appendices, worksheets, etc.) as well as items which you will need multiple copies of (e.g., assessments, clinician checklists) are available for download from the Treatments That Work website at www.oxfordclinicalpsych.com/ dementiacaregivers*

What is the ABC process?

We can think about challenging behaviors in terms of ABCs:

- A is for *antecedents*, or things that happen before the behavior.
- B is for the *behavior* we want to change.
- C is for *consequence*, or what happens just after the behavior.

Changing behaviors by changing antecedents

We can change antecedents by using *cues*. The following are examples of cues that may be helpful in working with persons with dementia. These cues can serve as antecedents to positive behaviors:

- *Visual Cues:* name tags or labels on familiar objects, gestures, larger than usual letters, underlined words.
- *Auditory Cues:* verbal reminder, bell, music, a door closing, a timer going off.
- *Tactile Cues:* a handshake, touch on the elbow, hug, or kiss.

Other antecedents that can help prevent challenging behaviors include:

- Keeping the care recipient involved in an activity can prevent wandering.
- Taking them to the bathroom at regular intervals can prevent accidents.
- Taking the knobs off the stove can prevent a burn or a fire.

Changing behaviors by changing consequences

We can change consequences by using positive reinforcement. We can reward behaviors we want to increase. Examples of reinforcements for desirable behaviors are:

- Giving the individual something they like: food, an object, attention, a smile.
- Saying something positive: conversing, praising, instructing, appreciating.
- Doing something kind: assisting, comforting, hugging.

Other consequences that can help prevent challenging behaviors include:

- Ignoring a bothersome behavior.
- Drawing attention away from an upsetting situation.
- Changing the way we look at the situation, resulting in a change of consequence.

Sections of the plan

A Challenging Behavior Action Plan is written when a targeted behavior, such as "repeated questions," is identified. The Action Plan has five sections:

Section 1: *Define the Problem*

Present the specific behavior in objective, behaviorally defined terms that are meaningful to the caregiver. Presenting the challenging behavior in specific, concrete terms helps both you and the caregiver to see the problem in the same way.

Section 2: *Goal of Action Plan*

Define the desired change in target behavior as the goal of the Challenging Behavior Action Plan, and present this in general terms such as reducing, increasing, or enhancing (e.g., reducing the burden of bladder accidents).

Section 3: *Signal Breath prompt*

Present standardized text to the caregiver to provide integration of the Signal Breath relaxation strategy with the Challenging Behavior Action Plan.

Section 4: *Strategies for preventing a challenging behavior from occurring*

Challenging behaviors rarely emerge in a vacuum. There are events in the environment that often trigger the target problem. These triggers are called antecedents because they occur before the target problem occurs. There are often things that the caregiver or other individuals in the setting do to trigger a care recipient's challenging behavior; however, the trigger might be something like the ambient temperature (too hot or cold) or even something internal to the care recipient, such as pain. Examples: Does the problem happen only at certain times (hunger related)? Only with certain people (grandchildren could be overstimulating the care recipient)? Could the problem be related to the way the caregiver interacts with the care recipient (multistep commands; approaching from behind the care recipient)?

Section 5: *Strategies for guiding how you respond during or after a challenging behavior*

The challenging behaviors might be triggered by a specific event or situation, but how the caregiver or other family members respond to the behavior (the consequences or what follows the behavior) could make the problem either worse or better. The caregiver's response can take multiple forms. Caregivers can have behavioral, cognitive, and affective responses to the target behavior. A behavioral response is defined by the actions that the caregiver takes. For example, if verbal abuse is the target problem, the consequence may be that the caregiver is arguing with the care recipient or cursing back when the care recipient curses. The therapeutic approach may have less to do with changing the care recipient's cursing and more to do with helping the caregiver respond in a nonargumentative way when the care recipient curses. This is often not as easy as it sounds and requires closely tracking the problem, providing feedback, and fine-tuning the Action Plan over time.

Often, the most appropriate strategy is to change the caregiver's cognitive/affective response to the target behavior. Cognitive restructuring techniques can be used to elicit a more benign appraisal response from the caregiver. For example, some memory-related problems (such as repetitive questions) might be resistant to change because cognitive deficits cannot be remediated. The caregiver can learn, however, to appraise these problems differently (e.g., "Remember that your husband has a memory problem and his confusion and repeated questions are not intentional; he is doing his best").

Another therapeutic consequence might be to involve the care recipient directly. For example, involving the care recipient in an activity when the target problem occurs, or getting the care recipient to talk about a happy event to stop a challenging behavior. These are ways of distracting the care recipient before the behavior worsens.

Guidelines

Guidelines for presenting Challenging Behavior Action Plans to the caregiver

- Orient the caregiver to the ABC approach to challenging behaviors.
- Discuss the criteria for what "success" would be for the caregiver (i.e., the goal): Read the problem definition aloud to make sure that you and the caregiver have a similar understanding of the problem.
- From time to time a caregiver may forget what was discussed in the previous session or may no longer agree with the definition of the problem. In this situation, discuss the discrepancy with the caregiver with the goal of bringing them back to the previously agreed-upon problem definition.
- Discuss what would make the caregiver feel better about this problem or what it would take for them to consider the problem "solved" (i.e., complete elimination of the problem versus management of the consequences of the problem). Make sure that goals are consistent with goals that were defined in previous sessions.
- Remind the caregiver that the intervention strategies listed in the Action Plan require new learning and frequent practice. Explain that the process will unfold over the next few weeks as you work together on these and other strategies.
- Explain what the program isn't (e.g., "I won't be asking you to try new medications or go out and buy a lot of things.") and what it is (e.g., "I'll be talking to you more about things like communicating better with [care recipient's name] and making changes in your living space to make caregiving easier.").
- Encourage the caregiver to be open to new ideas and strategies.

- Describe the working relationship with the caregiver as a partnership in which you will continue to work together to refine and reshape ideas and strategies.
- Reiterate that we do things this way because we have worked with many caregivers over the years and have found these strategies to work most often; remind the caregiver that many other initially reluctant caregivers have found success using these strategies.
- Acknowledge that changes may feel awkward initially because the caregiver and care recipient have a long history of interacting in certain ways. With practice, however, attempting these strategies will become easier.
- Assess the caregiver's understanding of the strategy and its rationale, as well as their acceptance of the strategy.
- Recap the strategy and ensure that the caregiver fully understands each strategy before moving on (e.g., "I just need to make sure I explained this correctly. Describe for me what it seems I'm asking you to do.").

Guidelines for soliciting feedback from caregivers

- Use open-ended questions to assess the caregiver's acceptance of and satisfaction with strategies. For example, "Tell me when you will use this strategy." "What will keep you from using this new skill?" "What are the potential benefits of using these techniques?"
- Avoid questions with yes/no responses (e.g., "Do you like this idea?").

Guidelines for negotiating with caregivers

- Attempt to get "buy in" from the caregiver by asking them to try each strategy for at least a couple of weeks.
- If the caregiver refuses to adopt a strategy, don't get defensive. Ask them to try it for one week: "I can understand you're not wanting to use this technique. Because we have seen this work with so many people, I want to ask you to try it first a few times over the next week."

- After further discussion with the caregiver, you may determine that some strategies are a bad fit for the dyad, or the caregiver may completely refuse to try a strategy. Acknowledge that the strategy should be eliminated and develop an alternative Action Plan.

Demonstration and role playing of strategies

- If feasible, you should conduct a demonstration and role play after discussing the strategies with the caregiver. Note that demonstration and role play may not always be possible.
- You should demonstrate each technique listed on the Action Plan. Some strategies may require a physical demonstration (e.g., how to move the care recipient's arm during dressing), whereas others may only require a verbal demonstration (e.g., "I want you to begin the dressing activity with the following statement, 'John, please stand up.'").
- Consider the following language, "Watching someone do an activity or skill is often the best way to learn. Please watch how I demonstrate the strategy. I will pretend to be you, the caregiver."
- Role playing is a more elaborate form of demonstration. It can be useful when a strategy is especially bothersome or challenging to the caregiver. Role plays require that you, the clinician, take on both the caregiver and care recipient roles. Likewise, ask the caregiver to play the role of the care recipient so that they can see what it feels like to be a recipient of the care.
- Set up the scenario. To introduce a role play, you might say, "This strategy may be a bit more difficult for you to use, so let's practice. First, I'll pretend to be you, and you will be [your care recipient]. Then we'll switch." Describe a specific scenario within which to practice the strategy.

Practice and provide feedback for each strategy

- Have the caregiver practice the strategies or skills outlined in the Action Plan. Here is language for you to consider: "Often it helps to have someone watch what you're doing so you can remember what works and what is difficult. Practicing with someone can really help you find ways to improve. Show me how you will carry out this strategy. Let's go straight through the whole thing and talk about it afterward."

- Provide feedback by highlighting good points and points that need improvement. "I really liked the way you [describe the skill performed appropriately]. I have some suggestions about how things might go better in a few places. Can we try those parts again and do something a little different?" (Return to specific steps with corrections.)

Make assignments and contract with the caregiver

- Make specific assignments: For example, instruct the caregiver to begin using the strategies immediately and to stick with it until the next session.
- You can encourage caregiver implementation by "contracting" with the caregiver. For example, engage the caregiver to commit to the activity a set amount of times between now and the next session. Emphasize that we know things need to be tried repeatedly and consistently for them to be helpful.

Provide words of encouragement and express commitment

- You should provide specific words of encouragement such as, "I know this is a tough situation, but I do think these strategies will be helpful. I'll be here to provide support and guidance."
- Remind the caregiver of the timeline, pointing out that you will be working with them over the next few months.
- Commit to revising the Action Plan until, together, you find at least one strategy that works.

- Behavioral strategies can take from two to three weeks to begin to show a positive effect.
- The more consistently the caregiver applies the strategies, the more likely it is for the Action Plan to work, and the faster a positive effect will be found. Consistency is the key.
- It is not unusual to find a temporary worsening of a challenging behavior when a new Challenging Behavior Action Plan is employed. It is important that the caregiver is prepared for this. For example, let's say the target problem is repeated questions. In the past, the caregiver might have given the care recipient attention after each question. The Action Plan could be to no longer provide attention, but to respond with a statement such as, "Look at the photo book of your grandchildren." Because the care recipient is accustomed to receiving attention, they might initially increase questions until the distraction intervention kicks in.

It is not common for an Action Plan to be stopped altogether; it is more customary to modify the Action Plan. In general, keep a Challenging Behavior Action Plan active for the duration of the intervention; however, there are exceptions:

- *Exception #1:* Persistent worsening of the problem. If the caregiver reports that the problem is "a little worse" or "a lot worse" during two contiguous sessions since the Challenging Behavior Action Plan was initiated, modify it significantly, or try a new strategy altogether.
- *Exception #2:* Caregiver resistance. This is a bit more difficult to define. You can expect some resistance from caregivers in doing Challenging Behavior Action Plans as a matter of course. You are asking them to do some things differently—and executing behavioral strategies in a consistent manner can be difficult. Thus, your job is to provide understanding and encouragement. Encourage the caregiver to persevere with the Action Plan. From time-to-time, however, the caregiver will present with marked resistance to conducting a particular strategy. In this case, the particular Action Plan should be stopped. This decision is often a judgment call made by the clinician. However, if the caregiver bluntly states that they do not want to attempt a strategy, try to develop an Action Plan that would be acceptable to the caregiver.

CHAPTER 7

The last treatment component of the REACH OUT program is to provide caregivers with enhanced emotional/social support and, if needed, support with instrumental activities. The latter entails helping caregivers obtain assistance from community resources for making legal decisions, managing caregiving tasks, and handling difficult situations. Another goal is to reduce problems with social isolation and to help caregivers maintain contact with their social network. It is often the case that the primary potential source of emotional/social support can be provided by family members, friends, and other caregivers. In terms of instrumental support, the goal is to help caregivers receive the assistance they need with both caregiving and noncaregiving tasks (e.g. shopping, transportation). Support for these activities will come from both informal sources, such as family, friends, and other caregivers, and formal sources such as healthcare providers and community services/agencies.

The social support risk area does not involve a detailed training module. If social support issues arise during the REACH OUT RAM—Risk Appraisal Measure (Form 2.1):

1. Use problem solving to develop Action Plans addressing the specific social support risk (e.g., to improve communication and assertiveness), and
2. Provide information and referral.

Examples of enhancing social support

If communicating with family members is identified as a risk/problem, you can design an Action Plan for improving communication skills. More specifically, you can create an Action Plan to help the caregiver become more assertive in asking for assistance from others.

If the Risk Appraisal Measure indicates that the caregiver is isolated and would benefit from spending time away from caregiving, you could develop an Action Plan for identifying a group of family members and friends who would be willing to provide care to the care recipient so that the primary caregiver can leave the house to engage in some activity. (This latter problem also can be addressed in the emotional well-being session; see Chapter 5.)

Information and referral

Provide caregivers with a Resource Guide that includes information about various resources, community agencies, and services available in their area. A listing of some national resources is included as part of the Caregiver Notebook (Appendix A). Space has also been provided for clinicians to add additional national and local resources as they arise in regards to specific caregiver issues. It is up to you to research and discuss relevant local resources with the caregiver and to help them add the necessary information into their Caregiver Notebook. Below are a few types of local resources that may be helpful to get started:

- Local Area Agency on Aging
- Local dementia care centers
- Meals on Wheels or other food delivery options
- Home health aides
- Transportation services

This chapter highlights and reiterates important clinical issues, REACH OUT materials, and roadblocks to success.

A few clinical suggestions

- During the first session, briefly explain the purpose of REACH OUT and provide an overview of the intervention process.
- If possible, schedule the first session for 90 minutes, so that you can complete the Risk Assessment (refer to Forms 2.1, 2.2, and 2.3 in Chapter 2 of this guide), prepare the initial Action Plans, and give these to the caregiver.
- Although REACH OUT is a protocol-driven intervention, it is no less important for you to develop good rapport with the caregiver. Spend the first 10–15 minutes of the first session encouraging the caregiver to "tell their story," of how they came to provide care for the care recipient and the effects the caregiving role has had on the caregiver (both good and bad). Showing genuine concern and empathy for the caregiver at this and all other contacts will help you establish the rapport needed for you to be most effective.
- Many family caregivers associate the term "caregiver" with paid caregivers (home health aides, nursing assistants, etc.). Thus, it is best not to use this term during your interactions with them. There are alternatives to the term caregiver, and the best term often differs regionally. Use the most frequent term in your geographical area. Examples of alternate terms include "care provider" and "carer." Also, the term "care recipient" can be perceived negatively by the caregiver. It is best to refer to the care recipient by referring to their relationship to the caregiver (e.g. "your husband" or "your friend").

> **Clinician Note**
> *Information to be provided to caregivers (some of the appendices, worksheets, etc.) as well as items which you will need multiple copies of (e.g., assessments, clinician checklists) are available for download from the Treatments That Work website at www.oxfordclinicalpsych.com/ dementiacaregivers*

- Action Plan templates (blank Action Plans; see Appendix B).
- Action Plan template worksheets. These are identical to the short-form Action Plans except that extra spaces are inserted into all sections of the form to allow you to have plenty of space to write notes, generate brainstorming ideas, note possible solutions, and so forth. These worksheets are not included in this guide (although Appendix C shows some samples). You can develop your own forms by inserting additional lines on the template with word processing software. After you and the caregiver have decided on an Action Plan, summarize the plan and write it out in detail on the Action Plan template.
- Remember, it is critical for you to give the original of the completed Action Plan to the caregiver and to keep a copy for yourself. A copy can be made with either a portable scanner or by taking a photo of the document with a smartphone. Although not required, there are smartphone applications available to help label and organize these documents. In our research, we have used the Tiny Scanner Application on an iPhone. The REACH OUT Clinician Treatment Implementation and Tracking Checklists (Appendix J) also can be used to monitor treatment implementation and to track progress. Form J.1 is used to track fidelity to the original protocol and Form J.2 is used on a session-by-session basis to note subjective impressions and caregiver progress.

Overcoming barriers

Table 8.1 contains a list of common problems that you may encounter as well as some potential solutions.

Table 8.1. Common Barriers and Solutions

Problem	Possible Solution
Caregiver wants to show you pictures or mementos from the past	Spend a few minutes on this, and then gently redirect. Do not "cut them off." This can negatively impact rapport.
Caregiver repeatedly brings up problems that have nothing to do with the intervention agenda	Refocus the caregiver. Remind them that you have a limited amount of time to meet and that you want to make the most of your time together. If the problem continues, consider setting an agenda with the caregiver. For example, spend the first 10 minutes of the meeting catching up on the week's events and the remaining time on the goal of the session. Share this agenda with the caregiver.
Caregiver reports that a crisis occurred during the week	Assess and evaluate the caregiver's care crisis. Follow adverse events protocol as applicable. In Appendix I, we present some common adverse events encountered during treatment sessions. If not a "crisis," refocus the caregiver or use applicable Action Plan.
Caregiver is not interested in the topic or does not want to continue topic	Encourage the caregiver to try the topic for a short period as an experiment to test it out; remind them that it has been helpful for many caregivers. Help the caregiver express concerns about the topic and identify barriers. Use the problem-solving strategy to find a solution.
Caregiver reports, "I am not making progress"	Remind the caregiver that progress is often slow and comes in small steps. The more the caregiver practices the more progress they will see.
Caregiver visual/hearing impairment requires changes to protocol	Increase font size of essential material/homework and discuss recording of essential material if appropriate. Minimize noise and discuss amplification options if available. Frequently ask caregiver to repeat their understanding of material.
Caregiver reading/literacy level/ understanding of English is low	Revise material to three key points per session. Use familiar/simple words. Consider recording key points and having caregiver record home practice where appropriate. Ask caregiver to repeat back their understanding of the material.

The REACH OUT Caregiver Support Program

Caregiver Notebook

Your Caregiver Notebook will serve a very important purpose while you are in The REACH OUT Program. Your clinician will refer to the items found in your notebook during sessions and will also encourage you to read through the notebook on your own.

Table of Contents

1. **Alzheimer's Disease and Caregiving**
   - About Alzheimer's disease and related dementias
   - Caregiver Guide
2. **Safety Information**
   - Home Safety for People with Alzheimer's disease
   - Smoking Fact Sheet
   - Wandering Fact Sheet
3. **Healthy Lifestyle Guide**
4. **Stress and Relaxation**
   - Some Effects of Stress
   - Steps You Can Take to Reduce Stress
   - Signal Breath Relaxation
5. **Caregiving Challenges**
   - Visiting
   - Advance Care Planning
6. **National and Local Resources**

Notes

1. Alzheimer's Disease and Caregiving

Most people with a loved one who has been diagnosed with Alzheimer's disease have many questions about the disease. In this section, you will find informative materials about memory loss, Alzheimer's disease, and dementia. In addition, you will find information regarding caregiving. These materials will help you understand the disease and your role in caring for your loved one, and provide an idea of what to expect as the disease progresses.

Materials included in this section are:

About Alzheimer's Disease

This booklet can be downloaded at: https://order.nia.nih.gov/publication/understanding-alzheimers-disease-what-you-need-to-know-easy-to-read-booklet

Caring for a Person with Alzheimer's Disease

Your Easy-to-Use Guide: Get Alzheimer's caregiving information and advice in this comprehensive, easy-to-read guide. Learn caregiving tips, safety information, common medical problems, and how to care for yourself. This booklet can be downloaded at: https://order.nia.nih.gov/publication/caring-for-a-person-with-alzheimers-disease-your-easy-to-use-guide

2. Safety Information

Some symptoms of Alzheimer's disease such as wandering, confusion, and forgetfulness will make it necessary for you to take a new look around your home and surrounding areas. You will want to make sure your loved one is safe and secure in and around your home. Your clinician will help you with this task.

In this section, you will find informative materials about the following:

- the importance of smoke detectors,
- securing all potentially dangerous substances and objects,
- the importance of identification bracelets or other forms of identification,
- monitoring all smoking by your loved one,
- kitchen safety,
- basic supervision guidelines,
- wandering risks, and
- the dangers of allowing your loved one to drive.

Materials included in this section are:

- *Home Safety for People with Alzheimer's Disease*
- *Smoking Fact Sheet*
- *Wandering Fact Sheet*

Home Safety for People with Alzheimer's Disease

In the kitchen and bathroom

- Make the stove safe. Some electric stoves have a switch in the back that will make it impossible to turn the stove on. You can remove the knobs from gas or electric stoves or buy protective covers for knobs and burners.
- Unplug electrical appliances that remain in view, especially at night.
- Paint or otherwise mark hot water faucets to minimize confusion. Lower temperature of hot water heater to a safe level.
- Keep a working fire extinguisher in the kitchen.
- Put matches, lighters, and poisonous cleaners out of sight and reach.
- Cabinets may be secured by the plastic lock mechanisms people use to keep toddlers out of harm's way. Also, put knives behind secured cabinet doors.
- Have working smoke detectors in the house.
- Disable the lock on the inside of bathroom doors.
- Use nonslip strips in the tub and showers and use bathmats with nonskid backing.
- Install safety bars in bathroom.

Other living areas

- Do not have any weapons available.
- Obstruct hot surfaces such as radiators.
- Know and practice a fire escape route.
- Have adequate but not glaring lighting. Use night lights for safety.
- Stairs are dangerous! Use a "baby gate" at top and bottom and be sure stair rails are secure.
- Remove all clutter from steps.
- Secure all doors, including basement and back doors. You can set up an alarm system to alert you when they are opened. You can place locks very high or very low.
- It might be appropriate to lock windows or use guards that lock the window open at a safe height.
- Clear floors of clutter. Secure rugs from slipping or remove them.
- Placing reflector tape on places where the care recipient bumps into things can help. Rubber soles on shoes and slippers are less likely to slip.
- Remove poisonous houseplants.
- Have emergency numbers available by each phone. Include police, fire department, doctors' names and numbers, poison control center, and nearest reliable neighbor. Remember 911.
- Buy or prepare a first aid kit.

Smoking Fact Sheet

If your relative smokes cigarettes, cigars, or pipes alone in the home, there can be cause for worry. Smoking creates the potential for danger because lit cigarettes, pipes, or cigars can be forgotten or dropped in the house. Cigarettes do not burn out; think of them as a lit match when you're considering safety. Someone who is confused also may try dangerous ways to light a cigarette—for instance, if matches cannot be found, they may try using the stove to light their cigarette.

Now is a good time for you to decide how you feel about your relative's smoking:

Do you want to help your relative quit?
or
Would you feel comfortable knowing that your relative smokes only when another person is present?

Steps you can take to help your relative quit smoking

Even though you may have wished for years that your relative would stop smoking, there are some simple methods that may help with smoking cessation:

1. Reduce your relative's desire to smoke.
   - Try a combination of smoking cessation techniques such as a nicotine patch, gum, or plastic replica of a cigarette as a method of occupying your relative's hands and reducing the stress that may cause smoking.
   - Talk to your relative's doctor about prescribing some short-term medications for smoking cessation that could be used along with the nicotine gum, patches, or inhaler.
   - Do not serve as much coffee or cola, or any other beverage that your relative normally drinks while smoking. Substitute fruit juices or noncarbonated beverages.
   - Be aware of "trigger times" when your relative likes to smoke—for example, after dinner or while talking on the phone—and have specific strategies to change the situation. Suggest a walk after dinner or give your relative an item to hold (e.g., a pencil) while talking on the phone.
2. Remove visual reminders about smoking.
   - Remove any cigarettes, lighters, matches, or ashtrays from your relative's environment.
   - Store smoking materials (cigarettes, lighters, etc.) in a secure location out of your relative's sight. This will help create an "out of sight, out of mind" situation for the smoker, which might decrease the craving.

- Remove all knobs from the stove when not in use and place them in a "safe" location where your relative cannot find them.
- Change cigarette brands as a way of reducing your relative's pleasure in smoking.

Steps you can take to help your relative smoke only while someone is present

Taking smoking away from your relative could be like removing an old friend. Maybe smoking is one of the few pleasures left for your relative, and while you do not wish to eliminate it, you want the activity to remain safe. Nicotine may act as a calming agent for your relative. Here are suggestions that might help you allow your relative to smoke safely:

1. Create a "smoking schedule" for smoking breaks during the day.
   - Write down all the times your relative smokes for one week.
   - Show the calendar to your relative and let them work with you in organizing a smoking schedule.
   - Post the smoking schedule in a prominent place (e.g., on the refrigerator) and show it to your relative when the urge to smoke strikes.
2. Limit smoking to a safe place in the home (kitchen, balcony).
   - Sit together while your relative smokes and make it an enjoyable time for both of you.
   - Clear away any clutter (newspaper, magazines, dried flowers) around the location where your relative smokes.
   - Provide a large, stable, fireproof ashtray for your relative to use. Do not place the ashtray on the arm of a chair or any other place that is unstable.
   - Confine smoking to an indoor location; an outdoor location could be dangerous (flammable grasses, etc.).
3. Will neighbors, family, or friends give tobacco products to your relative?
   - Inform family and friends about the new "rules for smoking" that are being used with your relative. Explain the importance of having someone present when your relative is smoking.
   - Ask family and friends to support you in your caregiving and the new smoking etiquette that you have put in place.
4. Things you should do if your relative smokes (alone or with another person present).
   - Make certain there is a working smoke detector and fire extinguisher available for your use and your relative's use.
   - Post emergency numbers and information in a prominent place for people who live in the home and emergency personnel.
   - Secure the house in a way that still provides your relative with an exit they can use to get out in case of a fire or other emergency.

Wandering Fact Sheet

Wandering and Alzheimer's disease

Many people with Alzheimer's disease wander away from their home or caregiver. As the caregiver, you need to know how to limit wandering and prevent the person from becoming lost. This will help keep the person safe and give you greater peace of mind.

First steps

Try to follow these steps before the person with Alzheimer's disease wanders:

- Make sure the person carries some kind of ID or wears a medical bracelet. If the person gets lost and can't communicate clearly, an ID will let others know about their illness. It also shows where the person lives.
- Consider enrolling the person in the MedicAlert® + Alzheimer's Association Safe Return® program (call 1-800-432-5378 to find the program in your area).
- Let neighbors and the local police know that the person with Alzheimer's disease tends to wander. Ask them to alert you immediately if the person is seen alone and on the move.
- Place labels in garments to aid in identification.
- Keep an article of the person's worn, unwashed clothing in a plastic bag to aid search dogs in finding the person.
- Keep a recent photograph or video recording of the person to help police if the individual becomes lost.

Tips to prevent wandering

Here are some tips to help prevent the person with Alzheimer's from wandering away from home:

- Keep doors locked. Consider a keyed deadbolt, or add another lock placed up high or down low on the door. If the person can open a lock, you may need to get a new latch or lock.*
- Use loosely fitting doorknob covers so that the cover turns instead of the actual knob.*
- Place STOP, DO NOT ENTER, or CLOSED signs on doors.

---

* Due to the potential hazard they could cause if an emergency exit is needed, locked doors and doorknob covers should be used only when a caregiver is present.

- Divert the attention of the person with Alzheimer's disease away from using the door by placing small scenic posters on the door; placing removable gates, curtains, or brightly colored streamers across the door; or, wallpapering the door to match any adjoining walls.
- Install safety devices found in hardware stores to limit how much windows can be opened.
- Install an "announcing system" that chimes when a door is opened.
- Secure the yard with fencing and a locked gate.
- Keep shoes, keys, suitcases, coats, hats, and other signs of departure out of sight.
- Do not leave unattended a person with Alzheimer's disease who has a history of wandering.

3. Healthy Lifestyle Guide

As a caregiver, it is *very* important for you to take care of your own health as well as your loved one's health. Many people find if they keep track of healthcare issues by documenting them, it is easier to stay organized and better manage your health. Your clinician will provide guidance in helping you focus on taking care of your health.

A healthy lifestyle can help you manage stress. Certain activities may allow you to take time out from your demanding schedule. Taking time to pamper yourself may help you relax and enjoy life.

Things You Should Do...

Exercise

- Exercise has many positive effects on the body. It reduces tension. It improves overall physical health.
- As a caregiver of a person with dementia, you may find it hard to exercise. Finding time may prove challenging. Choose an exercise program that will be practical and fit into your busy schedule. Make sure you talk to your doctor before you start exercising.
- Exercise can range from aerobics to yoga. As a caregiver, you may find walking to be a good exercise. It may fit best into your routine. You need no major equipment other than good shoes. Walking can be done at any time and near your home. Some caregivers find walking at the mall enjoyable. The care recipient can walk with you or be pushed in a wheelchair. Do not worry about the care recipient's behavior when you exercise in public.
- You may not be able to take the care recipient with you to exercise. If not, consider having someone sit with the care recipient while you exercise.
- Exercise programs are available through most cable TV stations and online for those with computer Internet access.

Nutrition

- Eating balanced meals and maintaining proper nutrition is very important. Try to eat foods that are high in vitamins and nutrients. Avoid too many sugary snacks.
- Make sure you have plenty of fiber in your diet by eating fresh fruits and vegetables.

- Limit your salt intake. Avoid foods that are high in saturated fat and cholesterol. Make sure you get enough to eat.
- Drink plenty of fluids. Drinking six to eight glasses of water daily is usually recommended.

Sleep

- Getting enough rest is important. Make sure you are getting enough sleep every night. Proper sleep helps you think more clearly, handle challenges better, and function better. If you are having problems sleeping, consult your physician.
- If your loved one with dementia is keeping you up at night because of behavior problems, let their and your physician know the situation.

Ask for Help

- Give yourself permission to ask for help before you burn out. If you don't, you may not have anything left over for the care recipient. Rely on family, friends, social services, and support groups.
- Arrange for two or three breaks during the week. Don't rule out help for even short periods of time. Such breaks are still helpful.

Medical Care

- Go to your doctor for routine checkups.
- Keep scheduled doctor appointments.
- Take medications as prescribed by your doctor.
- Get your blood pressure checked and keep a record.
- Get your hearing checked.
- Get an eye exam.
- Have your teeth examined by a dentist.
- Get your flu shot every year.
- Get a pneumonia shot, if recommended by your physician.

Change the Scene

- Try to get out of your house as often as you can, even if only for a few minutes. A quick walk to the mailbox, a walk to smell the flowers, or a brief glimpse of the stars can provide a quick break.

Stay Social

- Try to arrange time to see family and friends. Call a friend if you are unable to get out of the house for a visit. A phone call can be a wonderful way to lift your spirits. Also consider inviting a friend over to visit you; or, if in-person visits are not feasible then video calls using a smartphone or computer are another way to stay connected.

Treat Yourself

- Be good to yourself. Treat yourself to a dinner, concert, or movie. Buy yourself something you have been wanting.

Listen to Music

- Consider making your own recording of music you enjoy; you can play this whenever you need to relax. Choose music you find calming and peaceful.
- Music that helped you relax in the past may help you again. It may remind you of the relaxed feeling you had the last time you heard the music.

Read

- Reading and escaping into the world of stories can be a useful distraction and can be very enjoyable.
- Reading short stories or magazines can be helpful if you only have a short time to read.

Take Hot Baths

▪ Some people find the jets of a Jacuzzi tub help to reduce tension. Sitting in a warm bath can also help you relax.
▪ Add some bubbles as a special treat.
▪ Heating pads and hot packs also help to relax muscles.

Watch TV and Movies

▪ Some people find that TV programs and movies provide a nice escape from reality and are enjoyable. You might like curling up on the sofa with a warm blanket and a bowl of popcorn while watching your favorite movie.

Take Part in Hobbies

▪ Spending time on a hobby can also be relaxing and stimulating. Hobbies can range from bird watching, gardening, or biking to knitting, baking, or stamp collecting.

Things You Should Not Do...

Drug and Alcohol Abuse

▪ Drinking too much alcohol, using illegal drugs, or overusing prescription drugs is unhealthy. Talk with your doctor about treatment options.

Smoking

▪ Smoking is unhealthy. Talk with your doctor and/or the American Lung Association (ALA) about stop-smoking programs available in your area. The ALA can be reached at 1-800-LUNGUSA (1-800-586-4872) or visit its website at www.lungusa.org.

4. Stress and Relaxation

Caring for a loved one with Alzheimer's disease 24 hours a day can be exhausting physically and emotionally. Many caregivers put aside their own needs to care for their loved one, leaving themselves at high risk for stress. As a caregiver, clearly you have a duty to your loved one. But *your* needs are also important, and you have a duty to take care of yourself.

The most loving and responsible thing you can do for your loved one is to stay as emotionally and physically healthy as you can while caring for your loved one. In this section, you will find informative materials that will assist you in better managing your daily stress.

Your clinician will teach you a simple stress reduction technique, which is a breathing exercise called Signal Breath Relaxation. It is important that you practice this strategy and use it on a regular basis.

Materials included in this section are:

- Some Effects of Stress
- Steps You Can Take
- Signal Breath Relaxation

Some Effects of Stress

Potential physical effects of stress

When a person is under stress, the body releases the primary stress hormone called cortisol. Cortisol is very important, because it organizes systems throughout the body (including the heart, lungs, and immune system) to manage the stressful event.

When a stressor continues for a long time, it can take a serious toll on the body's ability to function and may lead to many health problems. Because caregiving can be a long-term stressor, caregivers can be at risk for conditions such as:

- High blood pressure
- Heart problems
- Increased susceptibility to colds and flu

Potential psychological effects of stress

When left untreated, chronic or long-term stress can cause problems such as depression, anxiety, anger, and irritability. Some people feel that they do not have the energy to do routine tasks and wish they were somewhere else. Some people start to feel hopeless and helpless, cry often, and notice changes in their appetite or sleep patterns. They may feel exhausted and empty. In summary, stress can take away from quality of life by lowering a person's ability to experience pleasure and a sense of accomplishment.

Potential social effects of stress

A caregiver's friendships and relationships often suffer due to the challenges of caregiving. Forming and maintaining social support can relieve stress by giving you a chance to discuss your thoughts and feelings. It is common for caregivers to feel that no one understands what they are going through.

However, caring for someone with memory problems does not have to be a lonely experience. As behaviors and care needs change in the person with dementia, let friends and family members know when you need help or maybe just a break. Caring for a loved one with dementia is too big a job for one person.

Many local support groups offer opportunities to meet others who have similar experiences. You might say that you don't have the time for these kinds of things, but it is important for your health and well-being that you make time. Caregiver stress can lead to illness or burnout if you do not take steps to prevent it.

Steps You Can Take to Reduce Stress

Give yourself permission to take breaks, even for just 15 minutes at a time. Taking care of yourself helps reduce stress and keeps you healthier

- Take a walk or make time for other physical exercise and healthy physical outlets.
- Make time to spend with friends and family you enjoy.
- Call friends, neighbors, or family on the phone to stay in touch with others.
- It's still important to laugh! Remember and use your sense of humor. Listen to tapes, records, podcasts, television, or people that help you laugh.
- Talk things out with a friend or get professional counseling if needed.
- Learn and practice relaxation techniques.
- Maintain religious or spiritual practices that are important to you (e.g., attend church or synagogue, pray, read religious literature).

Try to solve problems as they come up rather than avoid them. Ask for help or let others help you

- Establish priorities and organize time more effectively. Let the small stuff go. Again, ask for help or let others help you.
- Stop running negative thoughts and attitudes through your mind; learn healthier ways of thinking about yourself and your situation.

Take time for your physical health

- Keep your own doctor, dentist, and other professional health care appointments.
- Take prescribed medications as suggested by your healthcare professional.
- Try to get enough sleep and rest. Talk with your healthcare professional and other caregivers about ways to get enough rest.
- Avoid smoking or relying on alcohol or drugs to feel better.

Signal Breath Relaxation*

The Signal Breath was designed specifically to help you when you are in the middle of stressful situations. We chose this simple but effective technique because caregivers often have limited time for themselves.

The great thing about the Signal Breath is that it only takes a moment and can potentially reduce a lot of tension. Also, it can be used anywhere, at any time, as many times as you want. In fact, you could even use the Signal Breath in a crowded room and no one would know.

How to do the Signal Breath:

1. Take in a deep breath and hold it for a few moments. However, don't breathe so deeply or hold it so long that it is uncomfortable. About two or three seconds is usually long enough.
2. Exhale slowly while at the same time saying calming words such as "relax," "let go," or "easy does it" to yourself. Also, while you are exhaling, let your jaw, shoulders, and arms go loose and limp.
3. Repeat two more times, feeling your level of tension drop a little more each time.

Remember that it is important to practice Signal Breath regularly. Try to practice the Signal Breath at least once each day. Some caregivers find it useful to practice when they are not stressed, because it helps reduce feelings of tension when stressful situations ultimately arise. You should use the Signal Breath, if possible, whenever you are in the midst of a stressful situation.

---

* *The Signal Breath technique was originally designed by Dr. Richard L. Hanson at the Long Beach VA Medical Center in his work with chronic pain patients and has been adapted for use with caregivers of persons with dementia by Jocelyn Shealy McGee, MSG, MA at the Palo Alto VA Health Care System.*

5. Caregiving Challenges

Caregivers will confront many challenging situations while in the caregiver role. Two such topics include behavioral challenges during visits, and more globally, worries about your and your care recipient's future.

Materials included in this section are:

- *Visiting*
- *Advance Care Planning*

Visiting

Visiting with family and friends is important for you. However, others may be afraid to visit you or invite you to visit them. This fear may be caused by a lack of knowledge about dementia. Friends and family may not know how to behave with the person with dementia. They may worry about saying the wrong thing to you regarding the care recipient. You may have to do some extra planning to keep up social contact with family and friends. With careful planning, you can help make visits comfortable and meaningful for you and your friends and family.

Here are some reasons you and others may find visiting difficult:

- You feel down.
- You may not feel as if you have enough energy.
- You may not have enough time to entertain.
- You may find it too difficult to take your loved one with you on visits.
- You may be afraid of how they will behave.
- Others may fear imposing on you.
- Others may fear being around the person with dementia.

How to Make Visiting Easier for You

Below are some ways to make visiting easier.

What to do when friends and family come to visit

- Friends and family may want to visit you but be unsure whether they should. They may feel uncomfortable asking if they can visit. They may think their visit will be an extra burden to you. Do not wait for friends and family to ask if they can visit you. Invite them instead.
- Let them know their support and friendship are important to you. Visitors probably do not know your schedule. They do not know the "good" or "bad" times of the day for your relative or for you. Tell them when the best time is for you to have visitors. Ask them to call you before they come.
- You should let visitors know what to expect. Let them know what it is like to be around the person with dementia. Let them know how they have changed emotionally, mentally, and physically. There may have been specific changes, such as incontinence, that could be

upsetting to a visitor. Mention these to the visitor ahead of time. The more information visitors have, the less nervous they will be.

- Some people may be afraid they will have to help with caregiving duties if they visit you. They also may fear being left alone with the person with dementia. Let people know you want a social visit. Let them know you do not plan on leaving them alone with the care recipient. Let your visitors know how they can communicate with your loved one. Tell them what they should say or do. The more information visitors have, the less nervous they will be.
- Talking with your visitors may be difficult if your relative is there. They may interrupt the conversation frequently. Also, you may want to discuss things with your visitors that you think may upset the person with dementia. You may want to try distracting your loved one with another activity. For example, try scheduling the visit during your care recipient's favorite TV program or during their daily nap. Another good time to schedule visits may be while your care recipient is at an adult day care program.
- Plan the visit so it fits the needs and personality of the visitor. Some friends or family may prefer sitting and talking with you and your loved one. Others may prefer to do things. You may want to plan simple activities such as lunch or a picnic.
- Visitors may ask you what they can bring you when they visit. Be ready to make some suggestions of things that would brighten your day. You might enjoy flowers, food, or a book.
- Try to be patient and forgiving with family and friends. Many people have a very hard time facing up to Alzheimer's disease and other forms of dementia. People you wish would support you may not.
- They may avoid you out of their own fear of the disease. Try not to take such negative reactions personally. Instead, tell them about the disease. Help them lose their fear.
- A visit with family and friends does not have to be perfect. A little planning ahead will help make the visit more enjoyable for you and your visitors.

What to do when visiting in the homes of others

- Try to arrange time to visit friends and family alone on a regular basis. Even if it is only for an hour, it may be refreshing for you to have time with others away from the person with dementia. Perhaps a friend could stay with your loved one or you could arrange for them to go to an adult day care program. At other times you may want to take them with you to visit friends and family. This is OK as long as they are able to enjoy the visits.
- Prepare your host for what to expect of the person with dementia. Tell your host about your relative's emotional, mental, and physical abilities. Let the host know about any special

needs ahead of time. For example, let them know if the person with dementia needs to eat at a particular time.

- Suggest activities in which your loved one can take part, such as short walks or watching a favorite show on TV.
- Try to keep the daily routine as much like the one at home as possible. For example, if the care recipient usually takes a bath before breakfast then try to stick to that schedule.
- It may be better for your relative if the visit is kept short.
- Take pictures during the visit and preserve memories of good times for yourself and for the person with dementia.

What to do if the visit goes badly

- Deal with your feelings and talk with someone.
- Leave the situation; don't wait for things to get "better."
- Remember good times and try to see humor in the situation.
- Find out if something "triggered" your loved one's behavior.
- Try visiting again at a later time.

Advance Care Planning

What is an advance directive? How do you set one up? Learn how to decide and instruct others on what health care you would want to receive if you were unable to speak for yourself. This booklet on advance care planning can be downloaded at: https://order.nia.nih.gov/publication/advance-care-planning

If your loved one is in the mild stages of dementia, resources regarding setting up an advanced directive may still be helpful for them. For people with greater impairment, however, a medical healthcare proxy in combination with their primary care provider can help determine the best course of action. Finally, it is becoming more common for caregivers and people without cognitive impairment to document the medical care they would want if they were ever to develop dementia. Information regarding specific advance directives for dementia can be found at: https://dementia-directive.org/

6. National and Local Resources

A critical component of the REACH OUT Intervention is to help you feel more confident in your ability to solve problematic issues as they arise. Increasing your knowledge of national and local resources is one way to help build that confidence. Below, you will find a list of some national resources that may be helpful. Your clinician may suggest additional national or local resources that pertain to your needs, and you can organize them here for future reference.

National Resources

- Administration on Aging (AOA)—U.S. Department of Health & Human Services: AOA National Family Caregiver Support Program Resource Room
  https://acl.gov/programs/support-caregivers/national-family-caregiver-support-program
- Aging and Disability Resource Center (ADRC)—U.S. Department of Health & Human Services
  https://acl.gov/programs/aging-and-disability-networks/aging-and-disability-resource-centers
- Alzheimer's Association—Alzheimer's and Dementia Caregiver Center
  https://www.alz.org/help-support/caregiving
- Alzheimer's Foundation of America (AFA) Education and Care, Caregiving Tips
  https://alzfdn.org/caregiving-resources/
- American Association of Retired Persons (AARP) Caregiving Resource Center
  https://www.aarp.org/caregiving/
- Caring.com
  https://www.caring.com/
- Family Caregiver Alliance, National Center on Caregiving
  https://www.caregiver.org/national-center-caregiving
- National Alliance for Caregiving
  https://www.caregiving.org/

Local Resources

To be inserted by your clinician:

Notes

The clinician should place the Action
Plans here.

Generic Problem-Solving Form: Action Plan Template

Define the problem:
Goal of Action Plan:
Action Plan for solving problem: 1.   2.   3.   4.
General information:
You are a dedicated caregiver and you are doing a great job. We understand that this problem can be very upsetting to you and are committed to helping you with this problem. We believe these strategies will help and look forward to working with you in the coming weeks.

Notes

Sample Challenging Behavior Action Plans

1. Action Plan for Bathroom Accidents

Define the problem:

The care recipient wets themselves about eight times per day.

Goal of Action Plan:

Reduce accidents to no more than one to two times per day.

Please remember that dealing with challenging behaviors can be stressful. The brief relaxation strategies will help you deal with stress when dealing with this problem. In particular, we recommend using the Signal Breath technique immediately before you use the strategies suggested in this Behavioral Action Plan.

Strategies for preventing a challenging behavior:

1. Start care recipient on a toilet schedule.

- Toileting should be a standard procedure first thing in the morning, after meals, and at bedtime. Create a routine. It would be really helpful if you could write down the times when your care recipient relieves their bladder.
- Take your care recipient to the toilet every two hours. If they don't need to go, say you will be back in one hour to check again.
- If your care recipient doesn't want to go, guide them to the bathroom using step-by-step instructions.
- Remember to approach them from the front and begin each routine by announcing who you are and saying something comforting. For example, "Hello dear, I am your spouse/child, [Name]. I want to help you go to the bathroom. Please stand up."
- Remember to use warm and friendly actions (e.g., smile, soft touches).

- Encourage your care recipient to perform the tasks and offer the minimal amount of help that is needed.
- Only keep your care recipient in the bathroom for 10 minutes if they do not use the toilet.

2. Dress your care recipient in manageable clothing.

- Keep the person's dress simple and practical.
- Instead of choosing clothing with zippers and buttons, choose easy-to-remove and easy-to-clean styles, such as sweat pants with elastic waistbands or Velcro.

3. If the problem persists, try using an adult brief or a "Depends" incontinence product before accidents occur.

4. Keep a record for at least one week of the times your care recipient is wet and dry.

- From this information, I can work with you to find a pattern. For example, if your care recipient is wet every four hours, then I will suggest that you take them to the bathroom every three and a half hours.

Strategies for guiding how you respond during or after a challenging behavior:

1. **Tell your care recipient in a calm manner that they should try to get all the way to the toilet before going to the bathroom.**

   - Giving them this type of feedback every time an accident occurs may make them more likely to get to the toilet in the future.

2. **Avoid showing your anger or frustration when an accident happens.**

   - This will only cause confusion and distress.

   - In a calm voice, announce who you are, and continue to prompt and announce each step to get your care recipient to change clothes.

   - It is the disease that makes the person not able to get to the bathroom, not that they are trying to be difficult.

3. **Help your care recipient retain a sense of dignity despite the problems with incontinence.**
   - Reassuring and supportive statements will help lessen feelings of embarrassment, and that way you will feel more in control of the situation.

Other strategies:

General information:

You are a dedicated caregiver and you are doing a great job. We understand that this problem can be very upsetting to you and are committed to helping you with this problem. We believe these strategies will help and look forward to working with you in the coming weeks.

Define the problem:

The care recipient eats infrequently and prefers junk food.

Goal of Action Plan:

The care recipient will eat more nutritious food during the day.

Please remember that dealing with challenging behaviors can be stressful. The brief relaxation strategies will help you deal with stress when dealing with this problem. In particular, we recommend using the Signal Breath technique immediately before you use the strategies suggested in this Behavioral Action Plan.

Strategies for preventing a challenging behavior:

1. **Offer nutritious snacks during the day.**
   - This way you can monitor your care recipient's nutritional intake; for example, serve fruit, peanut butter, and crackers.

2. **Serve smaller portions on your care recipient's dish.**
   - It may be too difficult to concentrate on eating a full meal.

3. **Use spices to provide a pleasant aroma in the home.**
   - Cinnamon and orange potpourri smells appetizing.

4. **Tell your care recipient it's time to eat.**
   - Don't ask if they want dinner, because this gives them the opportunity to say, "No."

5. **Keep the same place setting for your care recipient at each meal.**

6. **Use bold color placement and white dishes in order to contrast the plate for them.**

7. **Use assistive devices such as built-up utensils or scoop dishes.**

Other strategies:

Strategies for guiding how you respond during or after a challenging behavior:

1. **Recognize that your care recipient is not as active as they once were and therefore they don't require the same amount of food during the day.**

2. **Keep a journal of food intake.**
   - This way you can recognize the amounts of snacks that they are consuming.

3. **Discuss this with your care recipient's doctor.**
   - Some medications suppress the appetite.

4. **Present food items one at a time.**
   - Offer chopped or soft foods, or cut food into small pieces if chewing is a problem.

5. **Establish a calm and accepting atmosphere when eating.**
   - Do not rush your care recipient to finish eating.
   - Engage in calm and pleasant social interaction.

6. **Offer smaller nutritious meals more often throughout the day.**

Other strategies:

General information:

You are a dedicated caregiver and you are doing a great job. We understand that this problem can be very upsetting to you and are committed to helping you with this problem. We believe these strategies will help and look forward to working with you in the coming weeks.

3. Action Plan for Difficulty with Personal Hygiene

Define the problem:
The care recipient does not wash themselves on their own.
Goal of Action Plan:
Maintain cleanliness with caregiver's assistance.
Please remember that dealing with challenging behaviors can be stressful. The brief relaxation strategies will help you deal with stress when dealing with this problem. In particular, we recommend using the Signal Breath technique immediately before you use the strategies suggested in this Behavioral Action Plan.
Strategies for preventing a challenging behavior: 1. Remove objects in the bathroom that are not used on a daily basis.   2. Use products that are familiar to your care recipient. Keep replacements on hand.   3. Adjust the hot water heater to no higher than 120 degrees to avoid burns.   4. Use adequate lighting.   5. Put grooming items out in the sequence they will be used.   **Other strategies:**

Strategies for guiding how you respond during or after a challenging behavior:

1. Tell your care recipient, "It's time to. . . ." Do not ask, because this will give them the opportunity to say, "No."

2. Walk arm-in-arm with your family member to the bathroom instead of pushing or pulling.

3. Allow your care recipient to sit in a chair or on the toilet seat.

4. Do not talk to your care recipient if they need to concentrate on grooming tasks.

5. Engage in grooming/hygiene tasks at the same time every day.

6. Provide physical assistance with all electrical appliances.

7. Use short, one-step directions.

8. Allow adequate time for grooming/hygiene so your loved one does not feel rushed.
   - Provide praise and encouragement such as, "You look so clean and nice. Let's go for a walk and show you off."

Other strategies:

General information:

You are a dedicated caregiver and you are doing a great job. We understand that this problem can be very upsetting to you and are committed to helping you with this problem. We believe these strategies will help and look forward to working with you in the coming weeks.

4. Action Plan for Communication Difficulty

Define the problem:

The care recipient does not respond reliably to caregiver requests.

Goal of Action Plan:

Increase the care recipient's responsiveness to your communications.

Please remember that dealing with challenging behaviors can be stressful. The brief relaxation strategies will help you deal with stress when dealing with this problem. In particular, we recommend using the Signal Breath technique immediately before you use the strategies suggested in this Behavioral Action Plan.

Strategies for preventing a challenging behavior:

1. **Help your care recipient focus attention on you.**
   - Call them by name.
   - Stand in front of your care recipient as they are trying to communicate with you.
   - Gently touch their hand or arm as you speak, while maintaining eye contact.
   - You may need to use orienting information before trying to communicate. Identify yourself and others to put your care recipient at ease.
   - Reduce or eliminate distractions (e.g., turn off the TV) to allow them to focus attention on you and the situation.
   - Remain patient, allowing your care recipient time to finish their thoughts.

2. **Use memory aids.**
   - Use index cards to remind your loved one of daily activities that need to be done, such as brushing teeth or dressing.
   - Use a memory board (chalk board or white board) where you can write notes (such as a phone number) or jot down where you are going when you leave the house. You can also use this board to write the day and date, or to leave comforting messages.

Other strategies:

Strategies for guiding how you respond during or after a challenging behavior:

1. Use one-step instructions.

- Break each task into the simplest steps and give instructions one step at a time.

2. Speak slowly and say individual words clearly.

- Your care recipient needs extra time for their brain to understand what you are saying.

3. Be aware of the tone of your voice when you are communicating.

- Use soothing and warm tones accompanied by positive facial expressions (smiling and eye contact).
- Avoid raising your voice.

4. Use gestures to help communication (e.g., pointing, flat hand to indicate "stop," motion for "come here," and nodding or shaking head for "Yes" and "No").

5. Offer simple choices that can be answered with "Yes" or "No."

6. Do not argue and avoid trying to convince.

- It will frustrate you and your care recipient and make the situation worse. You cannot win an argument with a care recipient with memory problems.

7. Please consider the following:

- Adjust what you expect from your care recipient. Their communication abilities are related to the disease. Please understand that you will need to learn new ways to communicate.
- Don't expect these tips to be easy or to come naturally. You will need to practice these skills.
- Whenever communication problems occur, make a calming and comforting statement to your care recipient. Try to avoid looks of frustration and irritation.
- If your care recipient is having trouble communicating, try to delay the activity or event until another time. Consider saying, "Let's wait and come back to that thought."

Other strategies:

General information:

You are a dedicated caregiver and you are doing a great job. We understand that this problem can be very upsetting to you and are committed to helping you with this problem. We believe these strategies will help and look forward to working with you in the coming weeks.

Define the problem:

The care recipient asks the same question repeatedly.

Goal of Action Plan:

Reduce the occurrence of repeated questions.

Please remember that dealing with challenging behaviors can be stressful. The brief relaxation strategies will help you deal with stress when dealing with this problem. In particular, we recommend using the Signal Breath technique immediately before you use the strategies suggested in this Behavioral Action Plan.

Strategies for preventing a challenging behavior:

1. **Distract your care recipient from whatever may be triggering the question.**

   - For example, make their favorite snack; involve them in a pleasant event or conversation.
   - Remember that someone with memory problems cannot remember having made these statements or asking the questions.

2. **Remove items (mirror, remote control, picture, etc.) that may be triggering repetitive questions.**

3. **Keeping your care recipient busy and active may help prevent them from asking repetitive questions.**
   - Boredom can sometimes trigger this behavior.
   - Create a schedule of activities during the day.

4. **Use humor.**
   - Humor is a very effective form of gentle distraction.
   - Focus the source of humor onto yourself or a situation so as not to hurt your care recipient's feelings if they cannot fully comprehend the meaning of your wit.

Other strategies:

Strategies for guiding how you respond during or after a challenging behavior:

1. **Keep a running record of what works and what doesn't work.**
   - This may help you focus in on an object or event that is triggering these questions.

2. **Try to stay calm and be patient with yourself.**
   - Repetitive questions can be very frustrating for you.

3. **Ignore the repetitive questions.**

4. **If questions center around the day or date, refer your care recipient to the calendar or a memory board with the day and date posted.**

5. **A memory board also can be used to post information about appointments or reminders of your whereabouts and time of return.**
   - Refer your care recipient to the memory board instead of answering the question.

6. **Write the answer to questions on an index card that your care recipient can hold onto or place in a pocket.**
   - Refer to the card in response to the question.

Other strategies:

General information:

You are a dedicated caregiver and you are doing a great job. We understand that this problem can be very upsetting to you and are committed to helping you with this problem. We believe these strategies will help and look forward to working with you in the coming weeks.

Define the problem:

The care recipient swears, cusses, or says unkind things to the caregiver about 20 times per day.

Goal of Action Plan:

Reduce care recipient swearing, cussing, or saying unkind things to no more than three times per day.

Please remember that dealing with challenging behaviors can be stressful. The brief relaxation strategies will help you deal with stress when dealing with this problem. In particular, we recommend using the Signal Breath technique immediately before you use the strategies suggested in this Behavioral Action Plan.

Strategies for preventing a challenging behavior:

1. **Prevent frustration that may lead to anger and upset by trying to identify the source or trigger.**
   - Be sure to consider care recipient needs such as toileting, eating, pain management, and illness.

2. **Ensure that your care recipient gets adequate rest.**
   - Schedule challenging activities at a time of day when care recipients are most rested.

3. **Provide opportunities for your care recipient to get exercise (e.g., a daily walk).**

4. **Avoid situations with loud noise or too many people.**

5. **Try not to criticize your care recipient.**

6. **Try to recognize when your care recipient is becoming upset and allow them to express feelings.**

Other strategies:

Strategies for guiding how you respond during or after a challenging behavior:

1. **Always keep your voice soft and low and use calming words.**

2. **Do not argue with your care recipient.**
   - Avoid criticism and use reassurance.
   - Pay attention to your body language, because your care recipient may pick up on your anger and frustration.

3. **If possible, take your care recipient away from an upsetting situation (e.g., go to a quiet room, go for a walk).**

4. **Try distracting your care recipient with an activity. For example:**
   - Ask them to help you with a task.
   - Suggest taking a walk outside.
   - Take your care recipient for a ride.

5. **Engage yourself in an activity away from the situation. The best thing you may be able to do for yourself is just to disengage from the situation. For example:**
   - Work in the yard or garden.
   - Practice the Signal Breath.
   - Listen to relaxing music.
   - Call a friend.

Other strategies:

General information:

You are a dedicated caregiver and you are doing a great job. We understand that this problem can be very upsetting to you and are committed to helping you with this problem. We believe these strategies will help and look forward to working with you in the coming weeks.

Define the problem:

The care recipient wanders outside of the home.

Goal of Action Plan:

Eliminate occurrences of wandering completely.

Please remember that dealing with challenging behaviors can be stressful. The brief relaxation strategies will help you deal with stress when dealing with this problem. In particular, we recommend using the Signal Breath technique immediately before you use the strategies suggested in this Behavioral Action Plan.

Strategies for preventing a challenging behavior:

1. **Secure your living area. These suggestions will help guarantee care-recipient safety as well as your peace of mind:**

   - Have someone place hook and eye latches either very high or very low on your outside screen door. Ask the salesperson at your local home improvement store if they have these latches with a spring-loaded catch. This type of latch will make the hook and eye latch more difficult for your care recipient to open.

   - Hang sleigh or jingle bells on all doors to alert you. These bells are often so delicate that they respond to the slightest vibration.

   - Ask your local hardware or home improvement store about pins designed to lock your sliding glass door.

   - Place a pad or mat that contains a pressure-sensitive alarm, in front of doors or by the bed. The alarm is triggered when a foot is placed on the pad in an attempt to leave or get out of bed.

   - Purchase a mobility monitor that will sound when your care recipient moves beyond a certain distance.

   - Place a "Stop" sign on doors that lead outside.

   - Tell neighbors and police to alert you if your family member is found unsupervised.

2. **Schedule specific times during your daily routine to allow your care recipient to spend time outside under supervision. Your care recipient may become more agitated if they are not allowed to wander, so it is better to control the wandering instead of discouraging it.**

   - Add another 30-minute walk to your daily exercise routine.
   - Engage your care recipient in activities related to their previous routines and interests (such as gardening, visiting museums, and walking at the mall).
   - Take your care recipient for a ride in the car.
   - Ask a friend or neighbor to take your care recipient for a walk a few days a week.

3. **Use various forms of identification. These suggestions will help aid in identification in case your care recipient gets lost:**

   - Dress your care recipient in brightly colored clothing to assure they can be spotted from a distance.
   - Place sew-on or iron-on labels with their name, address, and phone number in clothing.

Other strategies:

Strategies for guiding how you respond during or after a challenging behavior:

1. Don't panic or rush out on your own when you can't find your care recipient. Call the police. If your care recipient returns and you aren't home, they may go out again.

2. Have a list of important emergency numbers as well as a recent photograph handy in case of a wandering incident.

3. Try to distract your care recipient when they tell you that they need to go work on something outside. Asking them to help you with a task might help distract them.

Other strategies:

General information:

You are a dedicated caregiver and you are doing a great job. We understand that this problem can be very upsetting to you and are committed to helping you with this problem. We believe these strategies will help and look forward to working with you in the coming weeks.

REACH OUT Home Safety Checklist

General Safety

__ Emergency numbers and address are posted by each telephone.

__ Telephones are located in each room.

__ Telephones can be reached from the floor in case of a fall.

__ Inside and outside door handles and locks are easy to operate.

__ Doors have lever-action handles instead of round knobs.

__ Door thresholds are low and beveled or there are no thresholds.

__ Windows open easily from the inside, but they have a secure locking system that can prevent someone from entering from the outside.

__ The water heater thermostat is set at 120 degrees F or lower to prevent accidental scalding.

__ Medications are stored in a safe place according to instructions on the label of the package or container.

__ Carpets and rugs are not worn or torn.

__ Small, loose rugs have nonskid backing and are not placed in traffic areas of the home.

Kitchen

__ The range and sink areas have adequate light levels.

__ If you have a gas range, it is equipped with pilot lights and an automatic cut-off in the event of flame failure. Your local utility service representative can check this for you.

__ The range is not where curtains might fall onto a burner.

__ If you have an exhaust hood for the oven, it has easily removable filters for proper cleaning. Clean filters as needed.

__ The kitchen exhaust system is internally vented, discharges directly outside, or discharges through ducts to the outside and not into the attic or other unused space.

__ Countertop space allows you to keep carrying and lifting to a minimum.

__ Kitchen wall cabinets are not too high to be easily reached.

__ Lighting of countertops is enough for meal preparation.

__ Oven controls are clearly marked and easily grasped.

__ Oven controls are located on the front or side of the oven, so that you don't have to reach over the burners.

__ A single-lever mixing faucet is used. This type of faucet controls both the hot and cold water flow with a single control.

__ Flooring is not slippery and has a nonglare surface.

__ When cooking, pan handles are turned away from other burners and the edge of the range.

__ When cooking, you do not wear garments with long, loose sleeves.

__ Hot pads and pot holders are kept near the range.

__ If you have a microwave, it is operated only when there is food in it.

__ Small appliances are unplugged when not in use.

__ Drawers and cupboards are kept closed.

__ A sturdy, stable stepladder or step stool is used rather than a chair to reach objects in overhead cabinets.

__ Grease or liquid spills are wiped up at once.

Electric

__ Appliances, lamps, and cords are clean and in good condition.

__ There are no exposed, glaring bulbs in lamps or fixtures.

__ All electrical equipment bears the Underwriters Laboratories (UL) label.

__ Outlets are located where they are needed in every room.

__ Electrical overload protection is provided by circuit breakers, fuses, or ground fault circuit interrupters (GFCI). GFCIs prevent electrical shock and are particularly important in areas where water is used, such as kitchens, bathrooms, and outside.

__ Electrical service has enough capacity to serve the house and is up to code. You can call your municipal electrical inspector or a reputable electrical contractor to check the wiring in your house.

__ Extension cords do not carry more than their proper load as indicated on the cord or appliance.

__ Electrical cords are placed out of the flow of traffic and out from underneath rugs and furniture.

__ Smoke alarms are present in the home and are in working order. One way to help you remember to change the batteries is to replace them on your birthday—don't forget to mark it on your calendar.

__ Light switches are located near the doors.

__ Shiny or glaring work surfaces are not used.

Stairways and Halls

__ Steps are in good condition and are free of objects.

__ Steps have non-skid strips.

__ Carpeting on steps is securely fastened and free of fraying or holes.

__ Smoke detectors are in place in hallways and near sleeping areas.

__ Sturdy handrails are on both sides of stairway and are securely fastened.

__ Light switches are located at the top and bottom of stairways and at both ends of long hallways.

__ Inside doors do not swing out over stair steps.

__ There is enough space in the stairway to avoid bumping your head.

__ Room entrances do not have raised door thresholds.

__ It is easy to see the leading edge or nosing of each stair tread while walking down stairs.

__ Stairways and hallways are well lit.

Living Room

__ Electrical cords are placed along walls (not on carpeting or under rugs) and away from traffic areas.

__ Chairs and sofas are sturdy and secure.

__ Chairs and sofas have full arms to aid in sitting and rising.

__ The light switch is located near the entrance to the living room.

__ There is enough space to walk through the room leaving clear passageways for traffic.

__ Furniture, which might be used for support when walking or rising, is steady and does not tilt.

Bathroom

__ The bathtub or shower has a nonskid mat or strips on the standing area.

__ Bathtub or shower doors are safety glass or plastic.

__ Grab bars are installed on the walls by the bathwtub and toilet.

__ The towel bars and the soap dish in the shower stall are durable and are firmly installed.

__ A single-lever mixing faucet is used, or you have faucet handles that are easy to grasp.

__ Bathroom flooring is matte-finished, textured tile, or low pile commercial carpet (no throw rugs or bathmats).

__ Bathroom has even lighting without glare. The light switch is near the door.

__ The bathroom door opens outward.

__ The bathroom has a safe supplemental heat source and ventilation system.

__ The outlets are ground fault circuit interrupters (GFCI) that protect against electric shock.

Bedroom

___ A lamp or flashlight is kept within reach of your bed. Check batteries periodically to make sure they are working and keep a spare package of batteries nearby.

___ A nightlight is used to brighten the way to the bathroom at night.

___ Plenty of room is left for you to walk around the bed.

___ You have an adequate-sized nightstand or small table for the telephone, glasses, or other important items.

___ There is a sturdy chair with arms where you can sit to dress.

___ You have wall-to-wall low pile smooth surface floor.

___ Your bedroom is located on the first floor of the home.

___ A telephone jack is installed in the room.

Outdoor Area

___ Steps and walkways are in good condition.

___ Handrails are sturdy and securely fastened.

___ Doorways, steps, porches, and walkways have good lighting.

___ Porches, balconies, terraces, window wells, and other heights or depressions are protected by railings, closed with banisters, closed with fences, closed with accordion gates, or are otherwise protected.

___ Hedges, trees, or shrubs do not hide the view of the street.

___ Garage doors are easy for you to operate, even when snow is piled against them.

___ The garage is adequately ventilated.

Healthy Lifestyle Guide

As a caregiver, it is *very* important for you to take care of your own health as well as your loved one's health. Many people find if they keep track of healthcare issues by documenting them, it is easier to stay organized and better manage your health. Your clinician will provide guidance in helping you focus on taking care of your health.

A healthy lifestyle can help you manage stress. Certain activities may allow you to take time out from your demanding schedule. Taking time to pamper yourself may help you relax and enjoy life.

Things You Should Do...

Exercise

- Exercise has many positive effects on the body. It reduces tension. It improves overall physical health.
- As a caregiver of a person with dementia, you may find it hard to exercise. Finding time may prove challenging. Choose an exercise program that will be practical and fit into your busy schedule. Make sure you talk to your doctor before you start exercising.
- Exercise can range from aerobics to yoga. As a caregiver, you may find walking to be a good exercise. It may fit best into your routine. You need no major equipment other than good shoes. Walking can be done at any time and near your home. Some caregivers find walking at the mall enjoyable. The care recipient can walk with you or be pushed in a wheelchair. Do not worry about the care recipient's behavior when you exercise in public.
- You may not be able to take the care recipient with you to exercise. If not, consider having someone sit with the care recipient while you exercise.
- Exercise programs are available through most cable TV stations and online for those with computer Internet access.

Nutrition

- Eating balanced meals and maintaining proper nutrition is very important. Try to eat foods that are high in vitamins and nutrients. Avoid too many sugary snacks.
- Make sure you have plenty of fiber in your diet by eating fresh fruits and vegetables.
- Limit your salt intake. Avoid foods that are high in saturated fat and cholesterol. Make sure you get enough to eat.
- Drink plenty of fluids. Drinking six to eight glasses of water daily is usually recommended.

Sleep

- Getting enough rest is important. Make sure you are getting enough sleep every night. Proper sleep helps you think more clearly, handle challenges better, and function better. If you are having problems sleeping, consult your physician.
- If your loved one with dementia is keeping you up at night because of behavior problems, let their and your physician know the situation.

Ask for Help

- Give yourself permission to ask for help before you burn out. If you don't, you may not have anything left over for the care recipient. Rely on family, friends, social services, and support groups.
- Arrange for two or three breaks during the week. Don't rule out help for even short periods of time. Such breaks are still helpful.

Medical Care

- Go to your doctor for routine checkups.
- Keep scheduled doctor appointments.
- Take medications as prescribed by your doctor.
- Get your blood pressure checked and keep a record.
- Get your hearing checked.
- Get an eye exam.
- Have your teeth examined by a dentist.
- Get your flu shot every year.
- Get a pneumonia shot, if recommended by your physician.

Things You Could Do . . .

Change the Scene

- Try to get out of your house as often as you can, even if only for a few minutes. A quick walk to the mailbox, a walk to smell the flowers, or a brief glimpse of the stars can provide a quick break.

Stay Social

- Try to arrange time to see family and friends. Call a friend if you are unable to get out of the house for a visit. A phone call can be a wonderful way to lift your spirits. Also consider inviting a friend over to visit you; or, if in-person visits are not feasible then video calls using a smartphone or computer are another way to stay connected.

Treat Yourself

- Be good to yourself. Treat yourself to a dinner, concert, or movie. Buy yourself something you have been wanting.

Listen to Music

- Consider making your own recording of music you enjoy; you can play this whenever you need to relax. Choose music you find calming and peaceful.
- Music that helped you relax in the past may help you again. It may remind you of the relaxed feeling you had the last time you heard the music.

Read

- Reading and escaping into the world of stories can be a useful distraction and can be very enjoyable.
- Reading short stories or magazines can be helpful if you only have a short time to read.

Take Hot Baths

- Some people find the jets of a Jacuzzi tub help to reduce tension. Sitting in a warm bath can also help you relax.
- Add some bubbles as a special treat.
- Heating pads and hot packs also help to relax muscles.

Watch TV and Movies

- Some people find that TV programs and movies provide a nice escape from reality and are enjoyable. You might like curling up on the sofa with a warm blanket and a bowl of popcorn while watching your favorite movie.

Take Part in Hobbies

- Spending time on a hobby can also be relaxing and stimulating. Hobbies can range from bird watching, gardening, or biking to knitting, baking, or stamp collecting.

Things You Should Not Do...

Drug and Alcohol Abuse

- Drinking too much alcohol, using illegal drugs, or overusing prescription drugs is unhealthy. Talk with your doctor about treatment options.

Smoking

- Smoking is unhealthy. Talk with your doctor and/or the American Lung Association (ALA) about stop-smoking programs available in your area. The ALA can be reached at 1-800-LUNGUSA (1-800-586-4872) or visit its website at www.lungusa.org.

REACH OUT Pleasant Events
Summary Form

My List of Pleasant Events

☺ ☺ ☺ ☺ ☺ ☺ ☺ ☺
1.
2.
3.
4.
5.
6.
7.
8.
9.
10.

My Pleasant Event This Week

The pleasant event I will be doing this week is: _____

_____

_____

I will do my pleasant event on the following day(s) and time(s):

Day	Time	(Circle)
Monday		am/pm
Tuesday		am/pm
Wednesday		am/pm
Thursday		am/pm
Friday		am/pm
Saturday		am/pm
Sunday		am/pm

To post where I will see it every day (e.g., *refrigerator, mirror, nightstand*).

List of Pleasant Activities for _____ and Me

☺ ☺ ☺ ☺ ☺ ☺ ☺ ☺
1.
2.
3.
4.
5.
6.
7.
8.
9.
10.

The Pleasant Event We Will Do This Week

The pleasant event we will be doing this week is: _____

_____

We will do our pleasant event on the following day(s) and time(s):

Day	Time	(Circle)
Monday		am/pm
Tuesday		am/pm
Wednesday		am/pm
Thursday		am/pm
Friday		am/pm
Saturday		am/pm
Sunday		am/pm

To post where we will see it every day (e.g., refrigerator, mirror, nightstand).

ABCs of Challenging Behaviors

[A worksheet for the clinician to use during sessions]

Probes for the ABC Process

1	What is the behavior?	Notes
	■ "Take a minute and describe what care recipient does."	
	■ Clinician: Listen for irrational thoughts, misunderstandings about dementia, and unrealistic expectations of the caregiver.	
2	Why is this behavior a problem?	Notes
	■ People react differently to behaviors. What about this behavior really gets to you?	
	■ What bothers you?	
	■ Why does this get on your nerves?	
	■ Can you list the reason(s)?	
	■ What effect does this behavior have on you?	
	■ How does it make you feel?	
3	How would you like this behavior to change?	Notes
	■ When would you consider the problem "solved"?	
	■ What would make it seem to you that it was better? ("tolerable")	
	■ What would make you feel better about this problem?	

4	Why do you think this behavior happens?	Notes
	▪ Do you see any causes or triggers?	
5	When does the behavior happen?	Notes
	▪ Time of day?	
	▪ Days of the week?	
	▪ When does the behavior begin?	
	▪ Can you recognize any cycles or patterns?	
	▪ What happens right before the challenging behavior occurs?	
	▪ Does behavior happen constantly?	
	▪ How often does the behavior happen?	
6	Where does the behavior happen?	Notes
	▪ Is there a unique place in the house?	
	▪ Does it only happen in certain places?	
	▪ Are there places where it does not happen?	
	▪ Have you changed the surroundings of your family member? If yes, did it get worse or better when this happened?	
7	Who is around when the behavior occurs?	Notes
	▪ Do other people help care for your family member?	
	▪ Do you care for other people? For children?	
	▪ Is the behavior influenced by other family members or friends?	
	▪ How do other people react to your family member's problem behavior?	
	▪ Are there any special sleeping arrangements?	

8	What have you tried?	Notes
	▪ What do you do when care recipient does this?	
	▪ Have you tried anything that hasn't worked?	
	▪ Have you tried anything that seems to help?	
	▪ How often have you tried doing that?	
9	Additional information	Notes
	▪ Has your doctor been told of this behavior?	
	▪ If yes, what has your doctor recommended?	
	▪ Does care recipient have hearing problems?	
	▪ Does care recipient have vision problems?	

Supplemental Material for Deciding Risk Priority

If Caregiver Does Not Identify Any Risk; for example, no risks identified during risk appraisal or caregiver indicates previously identified risks were resolved.

1. Use a general probe question, such as:
   - "Are there things that bother you about caregiving or things that you would like to learn about?"
2. If "no" response, then use more specific probes listed below until you receive a "yes" response, and then go to #3. If "no" response to all probes, go to #4.
   - "Are there things that bother you or things you would like help with related to your relative's behaviors or need for assistance with daily activities?"
   - "Are there things that bother you about friends or family, or not being able to take care of yourself, or daily chores?"
   - "Are there things that worry you about the safety of your family member?"
3. If "yes" response, revisit relevant item(s) on Risk Appraisal (see the forms in Chapter 2) and follow standard procedure.
4. If "no" response to probes in the first or second session:
   - Review general educational materials provided in Sessions #1 and #2.
   - Discuss support group participation or other means of social support.
5. If "no" response to probes in second or third session:
   - Review general educational materials provided in Sessions #1 and #2.
6. If "no" response to probes by third attempt (Session #3 or #4), then use one or more of the following probes and strategies:
   - "Part of this program involves helping caregivers learn different strategies to determine what works best."
   - "Would you share with me what works best for you in keeping your relative safe?"

- "How do you keep in touch with your family and friends, or how do you make time for yourself?"
- "How do you handle challenging behaviors such as repetitive questioning?"
- "How do you keep from feeling overwhelmed?"
- Use active listening and validation.
- When possible, ask caregiver to demonstrate what they do—then go to a relevant Action Plan, highlight other strategies, and suggest the caregiver may want to try these other approaches as well.
- Ask the caregiver if you can come back to the home to check in. If "yes," then repeat probes for #6 above.

If Caregiver Has a Problem That Is Not Identified on Form 2.1: The REACH OUT RAM—Risk Appraisal Measure or other forms

1. See if the problem fits easily with existing Action Plan items. If not, bring the problem back to the caregiver and attempt to prioritize another problem first.
   - "I understand this issue is very important to you, and I'm wondering if working on a different issue first may help us focus our attention on this problem later."
2. If problem does not fit or there is no relevant Action Plan, indicate to the caregiver:
   - "This is not part of the REACH OUT program, but I can help you find others who may be able to help."
   - Try to identify a relevant resource with whom the caregiver can follow up.
3. If problem is relevant to a support group, suggest that as a resource:
   - "I think you will find some help with this issue in your support group. Try using your support group as a resource, and I will check in with you to see if you are finding it helpful."
4. Refer caregiver to a local Alzheimer's organization, Area Agency on Aging, Department of Social Services, or similar organization.

A Problem Is Identified but Caregiver Chooses Not to Work on It

1. If problem is an Adverse Event, reference the Adverse Events Protocols outlined in Appendix I.
2. If identified problem is not an Adverse Event, then provide the appropriate educational material or Action Plan, but do not go beyond that.
   - "Here is some material that you may find useful. Please let me know if at any time you want to learn more about this issue."

Caregiver Identifies Too Many Problem Areas

1. Prioritize items, beginning with Adverse Events first.
2. Negotiate to help identify the most important area on which the caregiver is to work.
3. Refer the caregiver to a support group to obtain information about select problem areas.
4. Near end of intervention (last two sessions), provide caregiver with relevant educational material for remaining issues.

Determining How to Move on to the Next Problem Area

- Using your intervention notes (Form J.2 in Appendix J), evaluate the caregiver's progress on effectively using strategies and note whether the problem has been resolved. If no progress, move on to the next problem area. Periodically check in with the caregiver regarding the status of the problem.

Involvement of Other Family Members in the Intervention

- Other family members can be involved in an intervention session if this is initiated by the caregiver. Make sure to document other family involvement on the REACH OUT—Treatment Implementation Checklist (Form J.1).

Guidelines for Working with a Caregiver with Low Literacy or Limited English Proficiency

- Provide Action Plans using bullet points and minimal wording.
- Use more demonstration and review pertinent written materials in more detail.
- Provide the Caregiver Notebook (Appendix A).
- Identify other family members, friends, or neighbors who may be able to help read material, if appropriate.

Adverse Events

Adverse Events are situations that may require more immediate action by you, the clinician. The most common adverse events are discussed briefly below.

Abuse

Evidence of verbal and/or physical abuse by the caregiver directed toward the care recipient requires an immediate response by you. Situations of mild verbal abuse can be managed through Actions Plans that help the caregiver improve communication skills with the care recipient. If, however, the caregiver refuses or is not able to control their verbal abuse, contact Adult Protective Services. Any evidence of severe and continued verbal abuse or any physical abuse requires that you contact Adult Protective Services.

Caregiver Depression

If during sessions, the caregiver presents with depressive affect, we recommend administering a brief depression screener such as the Geriatric Depression Scale (GDS). A copy of the GDS is included at the end of this section. If the GDS indicates a score of five or above, this suggests the presence of clinical depression. You should discuss the seriousness of the statements the caregiver makes regarding their own mood. Devise an Action Plan with the caregiver as to the actions they may take to help alleviate their depressive mood. The Pleasant Events material presented in Chapter 5 and Appendix F was designed for this purpose.

Consider suggesting that the caregiver contact their primary care physician so that an antidepressant can be prescribed.

Caregiver Threat to Hurt Themselves

Discuss the possible ramifications of self-harm statements made by the caregiver and devise a plan of action with them regarding the seriousness of suicidal statements. Increase monitoring of the caregiver's statements and other ways to be aware of caregiver's intentions. Consider devising a behavioral contract with the caregiver. If they continue to make frequent statements regarding self-harm, ask for permission to contact the primary care physician.

Care Recipient Access to a Gun or Other Weapon

Devise an immediate plan of action for blocking the care recipient's access to these objects. If the caregiver refuses or is not able to block the care recipient's access, contact Adult Protective Services and possibly law enforcement.

Care Recipient Driving

Advise the caregiver to stop the care recipient from driving and educate the caregiver about the dangers of the care recipient driving. Local resources (e.g., the Department of Motor Vehicles) have materials that discuss driving and dementia in your state. You, the clinician, should add those resources and/or materials to the Caregiver Notebook (Appendix A) and encourage your caregiver to read the materials. Suggest that the caregiver hide the ignition keys from the care recipient and develop an Action Plan to deal with any adverse reaction from the care recipient.

Geriatric Depression Scale (15-item)

The GDS-15 is a 15-item short form of the original 30-item Geriatric Depression Scale.

A score of 5 or greater suggests depression.

Choose the best answer for how you have felt over the past week.

1. ARE YOU BASICALLY SATISFIED WITH YOUR LIFE?	Yes	No
2. HAVE YOU DROPPED MANY OF YOUR ACTIVITIES AND INTERESTS?	Yes	No
3. DO YOU FEEL THAT YOUR LIFE IS EMPTY?	Yes	No
4. DO YOU OFTEN GET BORED?	Yes	No
5. ARE YOU IN GOOD SPIRITS MOST OF THE TIME?	Yes	No
6. ARE YOU AFRAID THAT SOMETHING BAD IS GOING TO HAPPEN TO YOU?	Yes	No
7. DO YOU FEEL HAPPY MOST OF THE TIME?	Yes	No
8. DO YOU FEEL HELPLESS?	Yes	No
9. DO YOU PREFER TO STAY AT HOME RATHER THAN GOING OUT AND DOING NEW THINGS?	Yes	No
10. DO YOU FEEL YOU HAVE MORE PROBLEMS WITH MEMORY THAN MOST?	Yes	No
11. DO YOU THINK IT IS WONDERFUL TO BE ALIVE NOW?	Yes	No
12. DO YOU FEEL PRETTY WORTHLESS THE WAY YOU ARE NOW?	Yes	No
13. DO YOU FEEL FULL OF ENERGY?	Yes	No
14. DO YOU FEEL THAT YOUR SITUATION IS HOPELESS?	Yes	No
15. DO YOU THINK THAT MOST PEOPLE ARE BETTER OFF THAN YOU ARE?	Yes	No

Sheikh, J. I., & Yesavage, J. A. (1986). Geriatric Depression Scale (GDS): Recent evidence and development of a shorter version. *Clinical Gerontology*, 5(1/2), 165–173.

REACH OUT Clinician Treatment Implementation and Tracking Checklists

---

Clinician Note

Information to be provided to caregivers (some of the appendices, worksheets, etc.) as well as items for which you will need multiple copies (e.g., assessments, clinician checklists) are available for download from the Treatments That Work website at www.oxfordclinicalpsych. com/dementiacaregivers

---

1. Client Name or ID _____

2. Date (mm/dd/yyyy) ____/____/_____

3. Time _____

4. Session number (1 to 6)   Check-in phone calls

1	*Phone In person*	1
2	*Phone In person*	2
3	*Phone In person*	3
4	*Phone In person*	4
5	*Phone In person*	5
6	*Phone In person*	6

5. Duration of the session: hours: _____ minutes:_____

Form J.1
REACH OUT Treatment Implementation Checklist

The purpose of this checklist is to help clinicians see if they are "on track" or adhering to the treatment protocol. Make sure to complete this form after every session to help with organization.

Date:
Session Number:
Which of the following topics did you cover during this session? Please check off each item on the list when completed. **Introduction** ☐ Introduce the REACH OUT intervention and establish rapport ☐ Ask the caregiver to tell their story ☐ Provide education on dementia ☐ Check in with the caregiver at the beginning of each session as to how they are doing ☐ Provide an overview of each session's purpose and structure **Risk Appraisal** ☐ Complete Risk Appraisal measures (Form 2.1, Form 2.2, Form 2.3) ☐ Review Risk Appraisal Measure findings with the caregiver and jointly agree on priority area(s) **Caregiver Notebook** ☐ Introduce and/or review the Caregiver Notebook (Appendix A) or relevant sections from the Notebook ☐ Ask the caregiver if they have any questions about the Caregiver Notebook **General Problem Solving** ☐ Review Risk Appraisal measure findings with the caregiver and jointly agree on priority area(s) ☐ Identify/discuss target problem(s)—use active teaching techniques when possible (i.e., role play, demonstration) ☐ Conduct brainstorming session with caregiver ☐ Develop written Action Plan(s) with the caregiver ☐ Review and/or modify relevant Action Plan(s) and strategies with the caregiver, as needed ☐ Assess the caregiver's responsiveness and the usefulness of strategies; problem-solve any barriers

During Today's Session: Action Plans

☐ Write an original Action Plan?

☐ Modify a Sample Action Plan (Appendix C)?

☐ Fine-tune an existing Action Plan?

Problem Behaviors

☐ Review ABC Process

☐ Complete ABCs of Challenging Behaviors, if appropriate

☐ Write Challanging Behavior Action Plan

Safety

☐ Complete a home safety walk-through with the caregiver, or

☐ Ask the caregiver to complete the safety walk-through

☐ Address any safety Adverse Events/alerts (guns, driving, etc.)

☐ Review safety material

☐ Incorporate safety recommendations into an Action Plan

Health

☐ Address the caregiver depression alert, if applicable

☐ Review the Healthy Lifestyle guide in the Caregiver Notebook, if appropriate

☐ Write Action Plan for enhancing caregiver health

Social Support

☐ Discuss social support options

☐ Encourage use of social support, if appropriate

☐ Write Action Plan for social support

Well-Being Strategy #1—Relaxation

☐ Introduce and/or review Signal Breath

☐ Identify any barriers to practice

☐ Encourage use of Signal Breath

☐ Write Action Plan for relaxation (optional)

Well-Being Strategy #2—Pleasant Events

☐ Introduce Pleasant Events (Chapter 5, Form 5.1, Form 5.2, and Appendix F)

☐ Review and/or modify Pleasant Events for the caregiver

☐ Write Action Plan for Pleasant Events

☐ Encourage use of Pleasant Events

Session Closure

☐ Obtain appropriate closure at the end of each session

☐ Summarize session accomplishments and set date for next session

☐ Ask the caregiver to practice health/safety tips, if applicable

☐ Ask the caregiver to practice Action Plan strategies related to target problem(s)

☐ Provide support and encouragement to the caregiver

Final Session

☐ Discuss any final issues or concerns

☐ Review target problem(s) covered during intervention and strategies that worked

☐ Review Signal Breath and/or Pleasant Events that worked and validate use of these techniques

☐ Encourage ongoing use of available formal and informal support services, including respite care

☐ Encourage continued use of the Caregiver Notebook as a resource to address newly emerging problems or concerns

Form J.2
REACH OUT Treatment Tracking (Clinician Evaluation)

This checklist is a clinician "tracking form" to help clinicians get a sense of session-to-session progress for their caregiver. Make sure to complete this form after every session to help with organization.

Date:
Session Number:
Indicate Intervention Area(s): ☐ General Education ☐ Safety ☐ Health ☐ Well-Being sections (relaxation techniques, Pleasant Events) ☐ Problem Solving (self-care, communication, behaviors, etc.) ☐ Social Support ☐ Behavior Management *Add Notes (e.g., issues discussed, recommendations, time spent)
Did caregiver practice, read, or try previous suggestions? Indicate yes/no and date asked:
If caregiver was unable to complete Action Plan from the previous session state the reason below: ☐ Too difficult ☐ Unacceptable ☐ Not enough time ☐ Did not understand ☐ Did not read ☐ Other (describe)

Problem status compared to beginning of treatment:

Is this problem:

☐ A lot worse

☐ A little worse

☐ The same

☐ A little better

☐ A lot better

References

Alzheimer's Association. (2019). 2019 Alzheimer's disease facts and figures. *Alzheimer's & Dementia, 15*(3), 321–387.

Arthur, P. B., Gitlin, L. N., Kairalla, J. A., & Mann, W. C. (2018). Relationship between the number of behavioral symptoms in dementia and caregiver distress: What is the tipping point? *International Psychogeriatrics, 30*(8), 1099–1107.

Belle, S. H., Burgio, L., Burns, R., Coon, D., Czaja, S. J., Gallagher-Thompson, D., . . . & Martindale-Adams, J. (2006). Enhancing the quality of life of dementia caregivers from different ethnic or racial groups: A randomized, controlled trial. *Annals of Internal Medicine, 145*(10), 727–738.

Burgio, L. D., Collins, I. B., Schmid, B., Wharton, T., McCallum, D., & DeCoster, J. (2009). Translating the REACH caregiver intervention for use by area agency on aging personnel: The REACH OUT program. *The Gerontologist, 49*(1), 103–116.

Czaja, S. J., Gitlin, L. N., Schulz, R., Zhang, S., Burgio, L. D., Stevens, A. B., . . . & Gallagher- Thompson, D. (2009). Development of the risk appraisal measure: A brief screen to identify risk areas and guide interventions for dementia caregivers. *Journal of the American Geriatrics Society, 57*(6), 1064–1072.

Dassel, K. B., & Carr, D. C. (2014). Does dementia caregiving accelerate frailty? Findings from the Health and Retirement Study. *The Gerontologist, 56*(3), 444–450.

Kessler, A. S., Hendricks, D., Mock, G. S., Robbins, L., Kuar, H., Potter, J. F., & Burgio, L. D. (2016). Translating the REACH OUT dementia caregiver intervention into a primary care setting: A qualitative analysis. *Alzheimer's & Dementia: The Journal of the Alzheimer's Association, 12*(7), P802.

Luchsinger, J. A., Burgio, L., Mittelman, M., Dunner, I., Levine, J. A., Hoyos, C., . . . & Ramirez, M. (2018). Comparative effectiveness of two interventions for Hispanic caregivers of persons with dementia. *Journal of the American Geriatrics Society, 66*(9), 1708–1715.

Ma, M., Dorstyn, D., Ward, L., & Prentice, S. (2017). Alzheimer's disease and caregiving: A meta-analytic review comparing the mental health of primary carers to controls. *Aging & Mental Health, 5,* 1–11.

Roth, D. R., Burgio, L. D., Gitlin, L. N., Gallagher-Thompson, D., Coon, D. W., Belle, S. H., . . . & Burns, R. (2003). Psychometric analysis of the Revised Memory and Behavior Problems Checklist: Factor structure of occurrence and reaction ratings. *Psychology and Aging, 18*(4), 906.

Schulz, R., & Beach, S. R. (1999). Caregiving as a risk factor for mortality: The Caregiver Health Effects Study. *JAMA, 282*(23), 2215–2219.

Teri, L., Logsdon, R. G., Whall, A. L., Weiner, M. F., Trimmer, C., Peskind, E., & Thal, L. (1998). Treatment for agitation in dementia patients: A behavior management approach. *Psychotherapy: Theory, Research, Practice, Training, 35*(4), 436.

Teri, L., Truax, P., Logsdon, R., Uomoto, J., Zarit, S., & Vitaliano, P. P. (1992). Assessment of behavioral problems in dementia: The revised memory and behavior problems checklist. *Psychology and Aging, 7*(4), 622.